THE COMPLETE GUIDE TO

Christopher M. Norris

STRETCHING

3rd edition

LEARNING
RESOURCES
CENTRE

HAVERING
COLLEGE

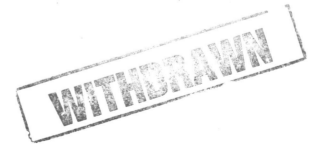
A & C Black • London

Note

Whilst every effort has been made to ensure the content of this book is as technically accurate as possible, neither the author nor the publishers can accept responsibility for any injury or loss sustained as a result of the use of this material.

First published in 1999 by
A&C Black Publishers Ltd
38 Soho Square, London W1D 3HB
www.acblack.com

3rd edition 2007

ISBN 9780713683486

A CIP catalogue record for this book is available from the British Library.

Typeset in Baskerville by Palimpsest Book Production Ltd, Grangemouth, Stirlingshire

Cover image © Getty Images
Inside photography © Grant Pritchard
Illustrations © Jeff Edwards

This book is produced using paper that is made from wood grown in managed, sustainable forests. It is natural, renewable and recyclable. The logging and manufacturing processes conform to the environmental regulations of the country of origin.

Printed and bound in India.

CONTENTS

ACKNOWLEDGEMENTS

My thanks go to Jan and Peter Bowen at the Alderley Pilates Studio for providing an excellent venue for the photo shoot. My thanks also go to Susie Gale, Victoria Jones, Jean Nadin, Madge Slater and Suzanne Hattersley, who modelled for the exercises, and to Grant Pritchard, who took the photographs.

PREFACE TO THE THIRD EDITION

The first edition of *The Complete Guide to Stretching* quickly became a well-thumbed book, striking a balance between science and practice which was popular with fitness instructors, practitioners and general readers alike. The second edition built on the first's popularity with an expanded theory section and double the number of exercises. New sections on fascial and dynamic stretching reflected the latest developments of practices that have now passed into common usage, making the book required reading for a great many practices, studios and other organisations.

This new edition fully updates the text, with a new chapter on Trigger Points and a number of new exercises. The illustrations and graphic representations are now detailed in full colour for the first time, and the exercises, both established and new, are accompanied by full-colour photographs, making practice and instruction an easy and beneficial experience for all.

Throughout the book, individuals are referred to as 'he'. This should, of course, be taken to mean 'he' or 'she' where appropriate.

Chris Norris

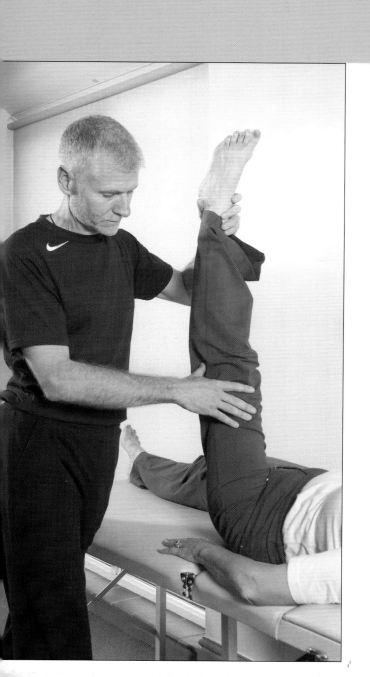

PART **ONE**

THE SCIENTIFIC PRINCIPLES BEHIND STRETCHING

BIOMECHANICAL FACTORS IN STRETCHING

The study of the effect of mechanical forces on biological materials is known as *biomechanics.* Biomechanical principles are important to all aspects of sports training, but especially to stretching. To be effective, and to prevent injury, stretching exercises must be applied on a foundation of good biomechanical principles.

Leverage

The limbs and spine act as levers when we move. A lever is simply a rigid bar that moves around a fixed point called the *pivot* or *fulcrum.* Two forces act on the lever, *effort* and *resistance.* The effort attempts to move the lever, while the resistance tries to stop movement. In the body, the effort is supplied by muscle contraction, while the resistance is weight. The weight is a combination of the weight of the moving limb and the weight of any object lifted. Take as an example the arm lifting from the side of the body (*see* fig 1.1). The fulcrum is the shoulder joint, the effort is supplied by the deltoid muscle, which contracts and abducts the arm, and the resistance is the weight of the arm.

How do you calculate the amount of leverage?

The amount of leverage produced in any exercise can be calculated by multiplying the weight of the resistance by the horizontal distance between the point where the resistance or effort

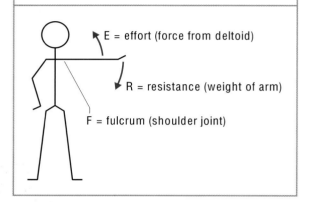

Figure 1.1 Leverage as the arm is abducted

E = effort (force from deltoid)

R = resistance (weight of arm)

F = fulcrum (shoulder joint)

acts and the fulcrum. Figure 1.2 illustrates a simple example of a lever. A resistance of 6 kg is placed 3 m away from the fulcrum. Multiplying these together gives a leverage force of 18 units. To balance this out, the effort has to be of the same magnitude. So, the 9 kg weight has to be placed only 2 m from the fulcrum for the lever to balance.

Leverage in stretching exercises

It is important to note that in the example given in figure 1.2 the horizontal distance between the fulcrum and effort or resistance is used, rather than simply the distance along the lever. This means that leverage will be increased as a body-part is moved into a horizontal position, and will reduce as the body-part moves away from the

Figure 1.2 Calculating leverage

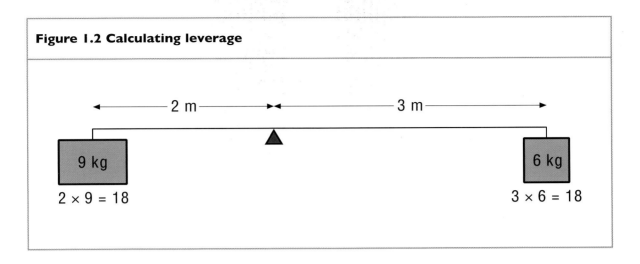

Figure 1.3 Leverage in weight training

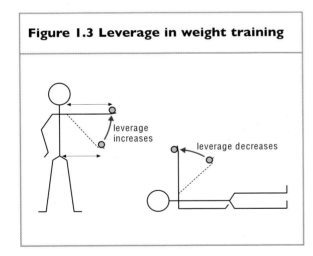

horizontal position (*see* fig 1.3). This fact must always be borne in mind when choosing starting positions for stretching exercises, especially with regard to injury to the spine. Take as an example a simple toe-touching movement. Performed from long sitting, the leverage on the spine is minimal (*see* fig 1.4(a)); however, the same body movement performed from standing (*see* fig 1.4(b)) places a considerable stress on the spine through leverage forces acting on the lumbar region.

This example illustrates an important safety factor with regard to leverage: exercises that involve moving the spine into a horizontal position will place great amounts of leverage on the spine and should be used with caution. Often, simply altering the starting position will move the spine away from the horizontal and reduce the stress on the lower back. When a horizontal position must be used, the spine should be supported. In the examples in figure 1.4, the athlete is stretching the hamstrings by bending forwards. This action places an excessive leverage stress on the spine. Simply by putting one hand down on the knee, the spine is supported and the stress reduced (*see* fig 1.4(c)).

Considering the effect of *gravity* is also important. In figure 1.5 the athlete is performing the splits. The leverage on the leg is excessive, tending to force the knee downwards, which opens the joint. This action can severely stress the medial ligament on the inside of the knee. Performing a similar action sitting down takes the weight away from the knee and, although the lever length is the same, the effect on the knee ligaments is considerably reduced, making the exercise far safer.

Figure 1.4 Reducing leverage by altering the starting position

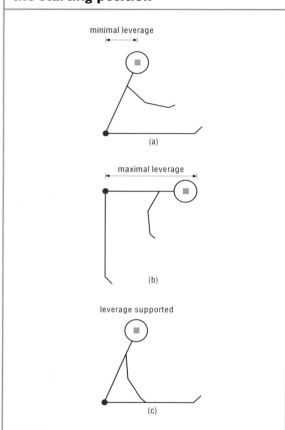

minimal leverage

(a)

maximal leverage

(b)

leverage supported

(c)

Key point: When devising a stretching programme, consider leverage and the effects of gravity. Are the exercises you choose using these elements to work with the body to enhance training or to work against it to increase the likelihood of injury?

Leverage and posture

Leverage is also important with regard to posture. A good posture (*see* chapter 5) is one that exerts minimal force on the joints and requires

little work from the muscles to maintain it. Anything that increases either *joint loading* forces or *muscle work* can increase the risk of injury and pain, and will certainly make the posture harder to maintain over a period of time. The human body, like any other object, has a centre of gravity, and the extension of this down to the floor is known as the *line of gravity* (*see* below). This can be thought of as the balance point of the body's levers. When a body segment rests on this line its leverage force is minimised, and when it moves away from the line the leverage force is increased. Take as an example the head resting on the neck (fig 1.6). In a good posture, the chin is held in and the centre of the head lies directly over the neck and the gravity line. However, if the head moves forwards – as it so often does when we are looking at a computer for a long time, for example – the leverage force is increased. Using the principle of calculating leverage we can see that, if the head moves forwards, it is as though it actually weighs more. A 10 kg head resting directly over the gravity line will only weigh 10 kg, but the same head resting 20 cm forward of this line will weigh 10 x 20, cr 200, units of leverage. This increased weight dramatically increases the forces on the neck and requires a significantly greater amount of muscle work to maintain it – so much so, in fact, that the muscles become tired and tight and feel knotted. The answer to this pain is simply to draw the head back onto the posture line by tucking the chin in slightly and thus reducing the leverage forces acting on the region.

Centre of gravity and stability

The *centre of gravity* of an object is its balance point, where all the weight of the object is focused. The centre of gravity of a symmetrical object, such as a brick, will be at its centre.

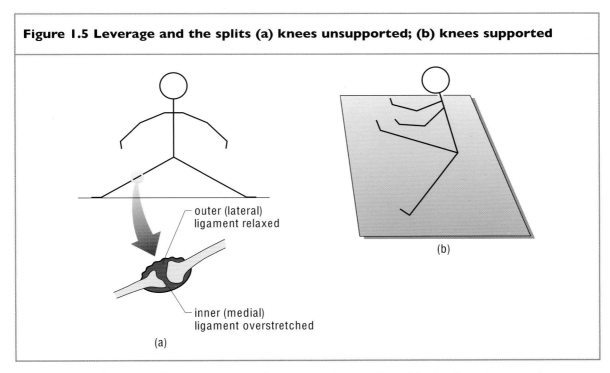

Figure 1.5 Leverage and the splits (a) knees unsupported; (b) knees supported

outer (lateral)
ligament relaxed

inner (medial)
ligament overstretched

(a)

(b)

However, in the case of asymmetrical objects, such as the human body, the centre of gravity will be nearer to the larger, and heavier, end.

Where is the body's centre of gravity?

Because the legs are heavier than the arms, when a person is standing their centre of gravity is not in the middle of the body at the naval, but lower down within the sacrum. As the body moves away from the standard upright position, the centre of gravity also moves. Lifting the arms overhead, for example, moves the centre of gravity upwards, while carrying something moves the centre of gravity towards the object being carried. In addition to the centre of gravity of the body as a whole, each limb also has a centre of gravity. For example, the weight of the arm will act through its own centre of gravity, which, rather than being in the middle of the arm at the elbow, is actually closer to the shoulder because the upper arm is heavier than the forearm.

What affects stability?

Extending the centre of gravity downwards towards the floor gives us the object's *line of gravity*. Where the centre of gravity is the

Figure 1.6 Leverage and posture

Figure 1.7 The centre of gravity

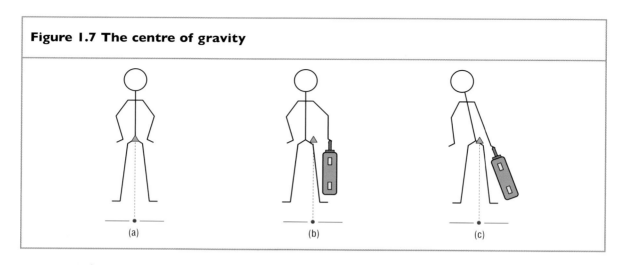

(a)　　　　　　　　　　(b)　　　　　　　　　　(c)

balance point of an object, the line of gravity can be imagined as a plumb-line hanging down from this point. For an object to remain in balance, its line of gravity must pass through its *base of support*. If the line of gravity moves outside the base of support, the object becomes unstable and will topple over. To compensate for this, the body position will change when something is carried. In figure 1.7(a), the centre of gravity of the body is within the sacrum. In figure 1.7(b), the suitcase carried in the right hand moves the centre of gravity of the body and case combined to the right. This would move the line of gravity outside the person's base of support, making him unstable. To compensate for this, the body position is changed by leaning over to the left to pull the line of gravity back within the base of support (*see* fig 1.7(c)).

Stability is an important safety factor when performing stretching exercises. An unstable position can cause an athlete to wobble or fall, unintentionally increasing a stretch and pulling muscles or spraining joints. When discussing stability, there are two factors to consider: first, the position of the object's centre of gravity; and second, the size of the object's supporting base.

A lower centre of gravity and a wider base of support will make an object more stable. In addition, the degree of stability is proportional to the distance from the line of gravity to the outer limits of the base of support. Take as an example a motorbike (*see* fig 1.8(a)). It has narrow wheels and thus a small base of support. In addition, the rider sits on the machine, so his centre of gravity is high. If the rider were to lean over when going round a bend, he would become less stable (*see* fig 1.8(b)). His base of support is the same, and his height above the ground is roughly the same, but his line of gravity has now moved closer to the edge of his base of support. The motorcycle-rider's position is much less stable than that of a racing-car driver where the car has a wide base of support (*see* fig 1.8(c)) and, because the driver sits low in the car rather than on top of it, the centre of gravity is lower.

How do you increase stability in an exercise?

The principles described above can be applied to the exercise situation. When performing standing exercises the centre of gravity is fairly high, so the feet should be apart to widen the

Figure 1.8 Stability, centre of gravity and base of support

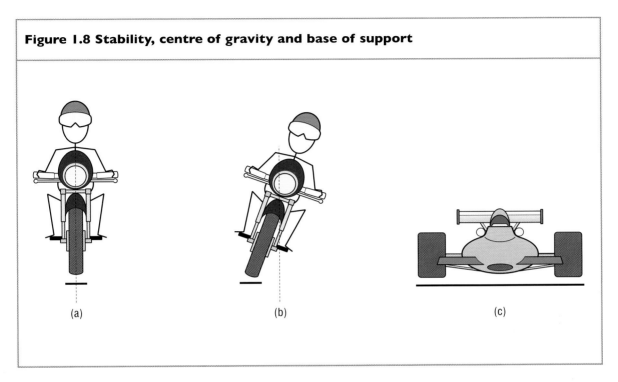

(a)   (b)   (c)

base of support, which will make the position more stable. In addition, bending the knees will lower the centre of gravity and further increase stability. When moving, the base of support should be widened in the direction of the movement, i.e. when swinging the arms forwards and backwards a wide stance should be taken with one foot in front of the other, and when moving the arms from side to side the feet should be astride. Fig 1.9 shows a variety of foot positions and their effect on stability. The narrow base (feet together) is less stable than the wider base (feet apart). In addition, where the wide base is lengthened in the direction of travel (lunge position, fig 1.9(e)), the exercise is more stable in a forward and backward direction but less stable in a side to side direction.

In fig 1.10 the yoga position known as the tree (page 143) is shown. The movement is basically a balance that stretches the adductor muscles of the hip on the bent leg. All three movements have a similar effect on the muscles, but the balance requirements are very different. In fig 1.10(a), the foot is placed on the shin and the hands are held by the sides, keeping the body's centre of gravity low. In fig 1.10(b), the foot is placed on the knee and the hands are at the chest, and in fig 1.10(c), the foot is over the hip and the hands are raised over the head. In fig 1.10(b) and fig 1.10(c), the weight of the leg and of the arms lifted above the head raises the centre of gravity of the body. The higher centre of gravity makes the position less stable and so it is harder to stay balanced.

Key point: When performing a stretching exercise, if you are unable to balance and find that you 'wobble', first, widen your base of support in the direction of the movement and second, lower your centre of gravity.

Figure 1.9 Changing base of support and stability

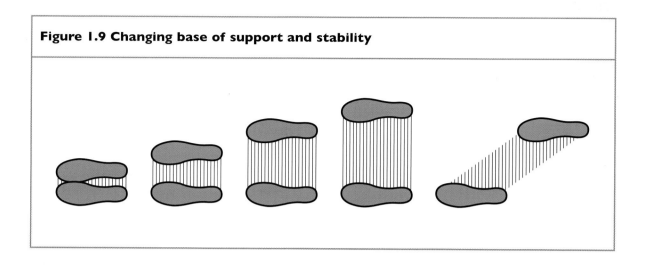

Figure 1.10 Stability in stretching exercises

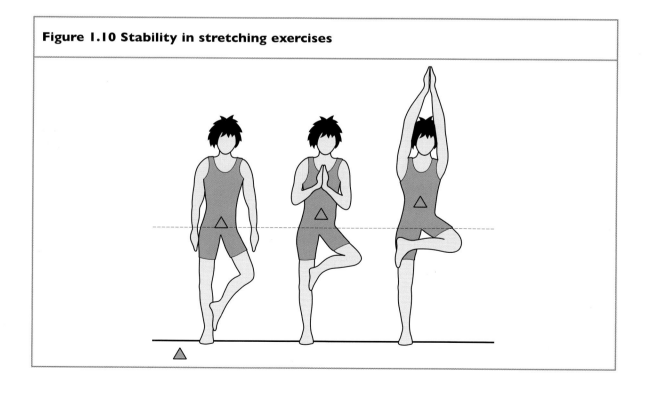

Inertia, friction and momentum

Inertia

Inertia is an object's resistance to change in motion, and is proportional to its weight or 'mass'. Inertia is the force that makes a car hard to push, but a bicycle easy. The heavier an object is, the more inertia it will have. Once inertia has been overcome and the object has begun to move, less force is required to keep it in motion. This is why a heavy object may need a 'good push' to get it moving, and then, as it starts to move, it does so with a sudden jolt and seems to 'run away with itself'.

A joint possesses a certain inertia due to the stiffness (viscosity) of its synovial fluid, and the extensibility of the tissues (ligaments and muscles) that surround it. The first part of any movement sequence will often be the most difficult because it is overcoming joint inertia. Once the movement is 'going', keeping it going is often easier. The first action in any set of stretches can be seen as a warm-up, and each subsequent movement will gradually increase in range. In addition, a warm joint will offer less resistance to movement in general, and its inertia will be less. A warm-up before stretching, or before any sport that involves range of motion exercise, is therefore important.

Friction

Friction, on the other hand, is the force that tries to stop one object from sliding over another. Frictional forces are the result of roughness on the surfaces of two opposing objects and can be reduced with the use of a lubricant like oil or water. On a rubberised floor, the roughness of the floor and the sole of the shoe produces a large amount of friction and gives considerable grip. A shiny wooden floor produces less friction, and a patch of water will reduce friction still further and may cause a person to slip and fall.

Momentum

Momentum is the combination of how heavy an object is and how quickly it is moving (mass and velocity). A heavy object, such as a leg or the trunk, which is moving quickly will possess a lot of momentum and will be very difficult to stop. The high degree of momentum can take over the movement so that the athlete is no longer able to control it: this is when injuries can occur. To reduce the likelihood of injury through momentum, rapid actions should only be performed in mid-range. When going to full range, actions should be slow and controlled to avoid damage to the joint structures and to muscles. Momentum is a particularly important factor in both dynamic and ballistic stretching (see Chapter 11).

Tension, compression and shear

Tension, *compression* and *shear* are all examples of mechanical stresses that can act on the body, causing the body tissues to deform.

Tension is a pulling force. When the spine is flexed, the spinal ligaments are tightened and subjected to a tension stress that causes them to lengthen.

Compression stress is the opposite to tension stress. It is a pushing force, applied along the length of a tissue. When a person is standing upright, the knee cartilages (menisci) take the weight of the body and compression stress is applied to them, causing them to flatten.

Shear stress occurs when opposite forces are applied to a tissue, causing one part of the tissue to slide over the other. For example, if an athlete who is running stops suddenly by digging their foot into the ground, shearing stress is applied to the knee. Body-weight tries to keep the athlete moving forwards, but – because the foot is fixed on the ground – the ground force pushes in the opposite direction. The result of these two opposing forces is shear.

Mechanical stresses and injuries

Both compression and tension stresses act in line with the tissue fibres, in the direction in which the tissues are strongest. Shearing stresses, however, are imposed at an angle to the fibres, making this type of stress potentially the most dangerous in terms of injury. For example, a fall on to a straight leg will exert a compression stress on the joint structures. These forces will be largely absorbed, unless they are very severe. During the fall, tension stress will be imposed on the muscles if the joints bend, and the elastic capabilities of the muscles will take some of the stress away from the joint. Falling at an angle will again cause some compression and tension, but shearing will also take place

between the body tissues and the foot and ground. This type of stress can cause injury, and a fracture may result.

Tissue reaction to load

The load–deformation curve

When a load is applied to a body tissue, the tissue will deform. The relationship between load (stress) and deformation (strain) can be represented graphically by the load–deformation curve (*see* fig 1.11). Initially, when the load is applied the tissue demonstrates elasticity. The deformation of the tissue at this point of the curve is directly proportional to the load that is applied (a relationship known as Hooke's law). As the load is released, the tissue returns to its original shape – it literally 'bounces back'. To begin with, the amount of deformation is proportional to the load applied and there is said to be a *linear relationship* between load and deformation along this part of the curve called the *elastic range*.

If the load continues, the tissue is stretched beyond its elastic range and a point is reached at which deformation becomes permanent. Past this point, known as the *elastic limit*, the tissue

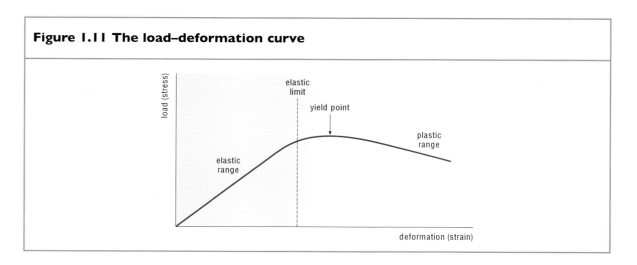

Figure 1.11 The load–deformation curve

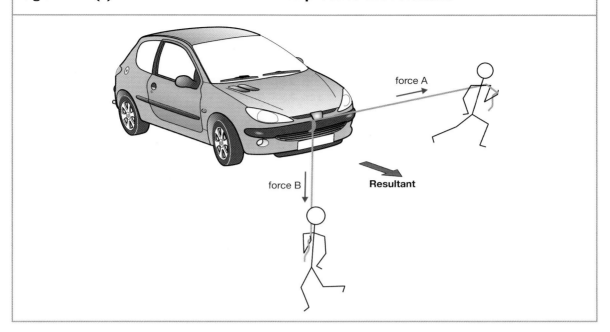

Figure 1.12(a) Forces A and B combine to produce the resultant

force A

force B

Resultant

will not return to its original shape when the load is released, and a permanent change will occur. Instead of acting in an elastic fashion, the material is now said to be *viscous* or *plastic* in its reaction to load. The more load that is applied, the more deformed the material becomes. Instead of returning the load and bouncing back, the tissue is absorbing and dampening some of the load.

Eventually, the yield point is reached, at the highest point of the curve. After this point the material continues to deform even though the load applied to it is not increasing; this means severe damage is occurring to the body tissue. This behaviour – continued deformation with constant load – is known as *creep*.

Properties of body tissues

Body tissues combine both viscous and elastic properties, so they are *viscoelastic*. One of the essential features of the deformation of viscoelastic materials is that it is time dependent. This means that when a load is applied rapidly (sudden stretch) the deformation will be elastic, and the tissue will spring back. If the load is applied for some time (stretch and hold) the deformation becomes viscous, and the tissue will slowly 'give'.

Composition and resolution of forces

Composition of forces

In figure 1.12(a), two men are pulling on ropes attached to a car bumper. Man A pulls at 45 degrees to the car; man B also pulls at 45 degrees but on the other side of the car. The net result is that the car rolls forwards. This process demonstrates the *composition of forces*. The forces

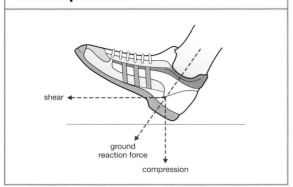

Figure 1.12(b) The ground reaction force has two components: shear and compression

the quadriceps muscles are pulling on the patella, the vastus medialis pulls inwards, and the vastus lateralis pulls outwards. The result is a centrally directed pull of the kneecap. However, if one muscle is substantially stronger or tighter than the others, the direction of the patella will change and pain may result.

Key point: When performing a stretch, do not just consider the actual movement that is occurring, but the forces that combine to produce it as well.

Resolution of forces

Where we have just one force, we can use the reverse process to obtain the two original forces which make up the resultant. Now we are using the process of *resolution of forces* to more accurately demonstrate the effect of the force on the body. For example, when someone who is running places their foot on the ground a force known as the *ground reaction force* is created. This acts obliquely to the ground (see fig 1.12(b)). This single force may be resolved into its two components: one of which acts vertically to create compression or

supplied by the men pull at 90 degrees to each other, combining to produce a third force – the *resultant* – which pulls the car forwards. If both of the original forces (called *component* forces) are equal, the car will move forwards in a straight line. However, if the right-hand force is greater than that on the left, the car will still move forwards, but it will veer off to the right.

A similar effect occurs in the body, where two muscles pull to create a third force. When

Figure 1.13 Patella compression can be very painful

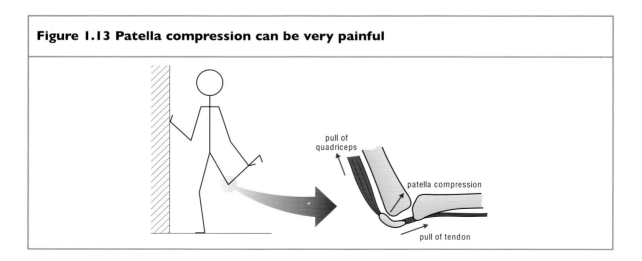

Figure 1.14 Axes and planes

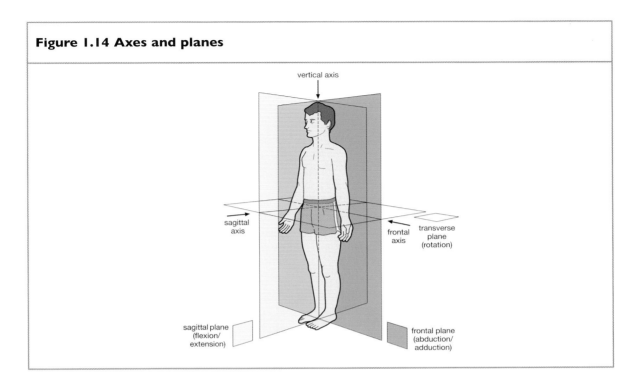

jarring stress on the foot; and one of which acts horizontally, causing shearing or friction on the foot.

Composition of forces in stretching exercises

The composition of forces can also be important when performing stretching exercises. Take as an example the quadriceps stretch (*see* page 97). As we bend the knee, the top of the patella is pulled upwards along the length of the femur and the patella tendon pulls downwards, in the opposite direction. The result is a composition of these two forces to create a third force compressing the patella on to the femur below. This action can be very painful in someone suffering from inflammation of the front of the knee (*see* fig 1.13).

Describing body movement

Axes and planes

For descriptive purposes the human body may be divided into three planes. The *sagittal* plane passes through the body from front to back, dividing it into right and left halves. The *frontal* plane divides the body into anterior and posterior sections, and lies at right angles to the sagittal plane. The *transverse* plane divides the body into upper and lower portions, and rests at right angles to the other two planes.

Each of the three body planes has an associated axis which passes perpendicularly through it (*see* fig 1.14). Movement occurs in a plane but about an axis. Abduction and adduction occur in the frontal plane about an antero-posterior (AP) axis; flexion and extension occur in a sagittal plane about a transverse axis; and

Figure 1.15 Anatomical terminology

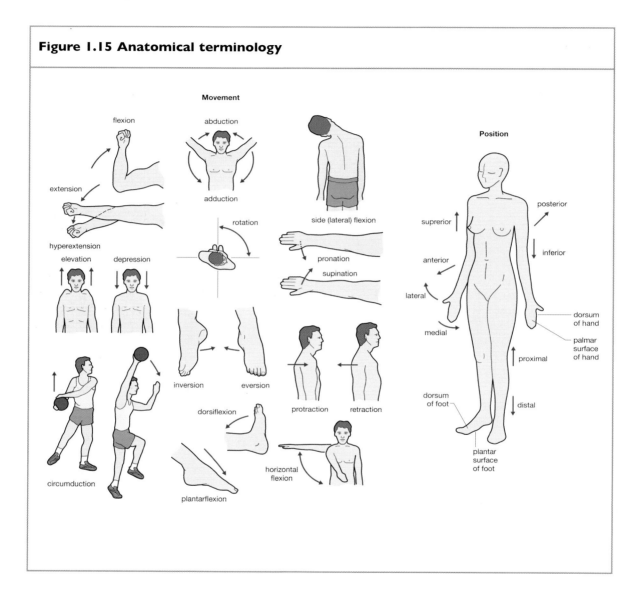

Figure 1.16 Range of motion

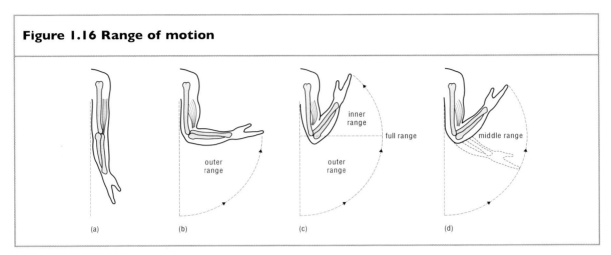

rotations occur in a transverse plane about a vertical axis.

In reality, movements do not just occur in one plane, but in several. This is because a complex series of movements links together to give a motion that occurs in all three planes about an oblique axis.

Anatomical terminology

Standard terminology should be used when describing body movements to avoid confusion. For example, instead of 'bending' we use flexion, and instead of 'straightening' we use extension.

To describe the position of part of the body, we again use standard terminology. So, instead of saying 'in front' we use the term anterior, and instead of 'above', the term superior is used.

Figure 1.15 shows the common terms used to describe movement and position of the body.

Range of motion

The *range of motion* (ROM) of a muscle refers to the length of the muscle at any point in a movement. *Outer range* is from a fully stretched position to the mid-point of the movement. *Inner range* is from this mid-point to a fully shortened position of the muscle. *Mid-range* is an area between these two extremes and is the region in which most everyday actions occur (*see* fig 1.16).

It is important that the body tissues are regularly taken through their full range of motion to maintain their extensibility and elasticity. When this does not occur, the muscle can shorten permanently, completely altering the function of a joint. For example, in a sedentary individual it is common for the hip flexors to become shortened, because most everyday movements only work these muscles within their inner range. The shortened muscle may then pull on to the lumbar spine, giving back pain.

Summary

- A lever is a rigid bar that moves around a fixed point called the fulcrum.
- Leverage is calculated by multiplying the horizontal distance between the fulcrum and

the line of action of a force acting on the lever.

- Keeping body parts close to the posture line reduces the effects of leverage.
- The centre of gravity of the body is near the sternum.
- When exercising, stability can be increased by lowering the body's centre of gravity (bending the knees) and widening the base of support (standing with the feet apart).
- As a body tissue is loaded, initially its reaction is elastic (it springs back) then plastic (it permanently deforms).
- Forces may be resolved into two components acting at 90 degrees to each other.
- Motion may be outer, mid-, or inner range.

JOINT STRUCTURE AND FUNCTION

Bones

The body has over 200 separate bones. Each is a rigid structure made from calcium, phosphorous and proteins. Bones may be divided into four major categories: long, short, flat and irregular.

- **Long bones** are the type found in the limbs such as the thigh (femur) and upper arm (humerus). Their primary use is to act as levers for the muscles to pull on when producing movement.
- **Short bones** are cube-shaped and seen in the carpels of the hand and tarsals of the forefoot.
- **Flat bones**, such as the scapulae and ribs, form broad areas for muscle attachment and serve to protect vital organs of the body.

- **Irregular bones**, such as the vertebrae, protect and support the body.

How do bones form?

Bone begins life as cartilage in the foetus. During the second month of pregnancy the cartilage bone begins to change into bone proper by a process known as *ossification* (see fig 2.1). This begins in an area in the middle of the bone known as the *primary* centre and gradually spreads towards the bone-ends. This central portion of ossified bone is called the *diaphysis*, while the end of the bone which is still made of cartilage is the *epiphysis*. During adolescence, a *secondary* ossification centre appears in the epiphysis. Ossification here spreads towards the shaft, leaving a thin cartilage growth plate (epiphyseal plate) sandwiched between the two regions of ossified bone.

Figure 2.1 Ossification of centres in the bone: (a) embryonic (b) infancy (c) adolescence (d) mature

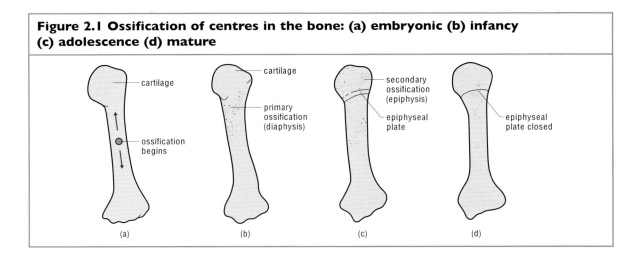

How do bones grow?

The growth plate is responsible for change in the length of the bone. As a person reaches maturity, the epiphyseal plate will disappear and the shaft and extremity of the bone fuse into one solid unit. The epiphyseal plate is an area of potential weakness in the young bone, and, if damaged, can result in permanent deformity of the bone. This is especially true of the upper part of the femur in sport, and great care must be taken when giving stretching exercises to children so that excessive strain is not imposed on the hip.

> **Key point**: When giving stretching exercises to children to work their muscles, consider the effects that these same movements are having on their growing bones.

What are bones made of?

As a long bone ossifies, its shaft becomes a cylinder with hard compact bone on the outside surrounding a central medullary cavity. The bone cavity contains bone marrow, responsible for making blood cells. The epiphysis is made from spongy cancellous bone with a thin compact bone covering. The other bone types do not contain a cavity, but instead are made up of a honeycomb of cancellous bone with a thin compact bone covering. This makes them light, although they may be bulky.

Joint types

In order for movement to occur in the body, the bones must articulate. The point at which this occurs is called a joint, and consists of two bones separated by various types of tissue. The shape of the bone-ends involved in a joint will dictate how much movement can occur, and which movement types are allowed. Joints may be broadly classified into three major groups, known as *fibrous* (immobile), *cartilaginous* (slightly mobile) and *synovial* (freely movable) (*see* table 2.1).

Fibrous joints

Fibrous joints allow little, if any, movement. Examples include the joints formed between the bones of the skull (a *suture* joint), those of the teeth (*gomphosis*), and *syndesmosis*, an example of which is found between the upper end of the fibula and the upper outer aspect of the tibia.

The edges of the bones forming the suture joints of the skull are jagged and separated by fibrous tissue. This type of joint will not normally allow any perceptible movement, and may close up completely after the age of 30. The syndesmosis is also separated by fibrous tissue, but contains more than the suture joint. The fibrous tissue in this joint forms a ligament that allows small amounts of twisting and stretching movements. The gomphosis consists of a peg which fits tightly into a socket and is held in place by a fibrous band.

Cartilaginous joints

In cartilaginous joints, the bones are separated by a pad of cartilage tissue, and both primary and secondary types exist. The primary cartilaginous joint has articular cartilage separating the bones. They occur as the growth plates at the ends of bones in children. At the beginning of adult life, the growth plate closes and the two pieces of bone (the diaphysis and epiphysis) become one bone. The secondary cartilaginous joints are found in the centre line of the body; examples include the spinal discs and the joint between the two pubic bones (known as the *symphysis pubis*). The bone-ends of the joint are separated from each other by a fibrocartilage pad, a structure which allows limited movement.

Table 2.1   Joint types

FIBROUS

suture
(skull)

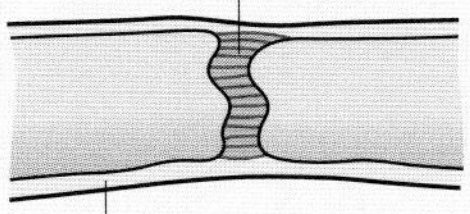

sutural
ligament
(fibrous
tissue)

periosteum

gomphosis
(teeth)

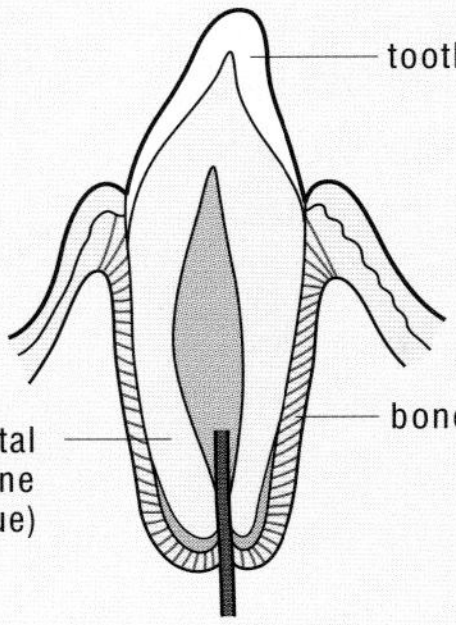

tooth

periodontal
membrane
(fibrous tissue)

bone

syndesmosis
(shin)

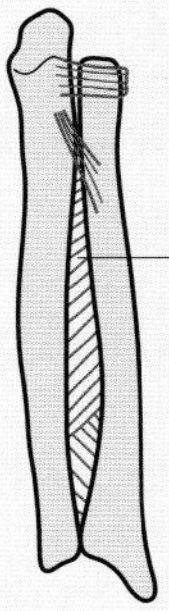

interosseous
membrane
(fibrous tissue)

CARTILAGINOUS

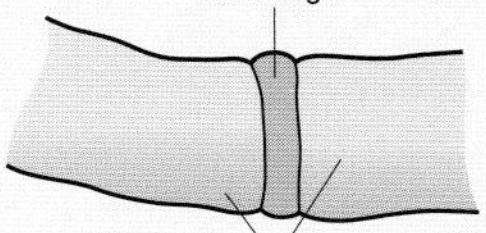

hyaline
cartilage

bone

primary (epiphysis)

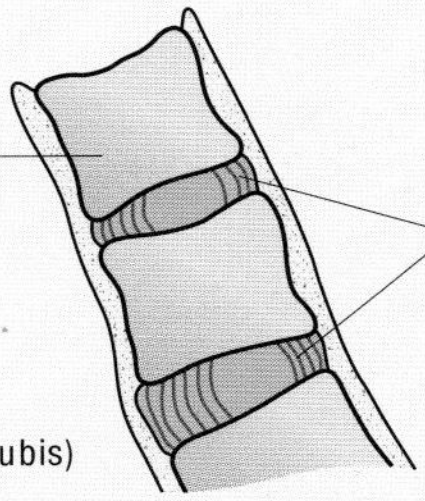

vertebral
(body)

intervertebral
disc

secondary (pubis)

SYNOVAL

plane (intertarsal)

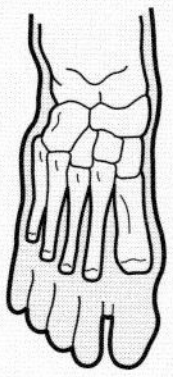

saddle (carpometacarpal)

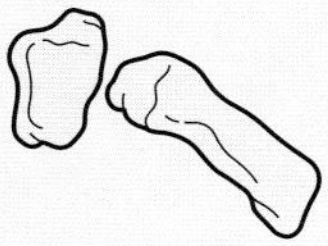

hinge (humeroulnar)

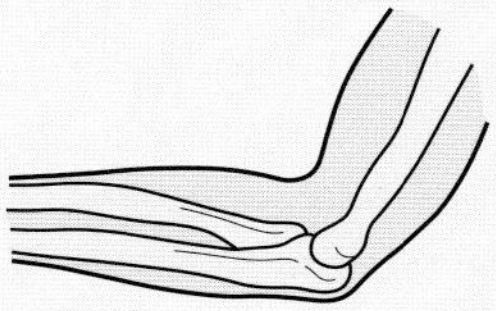

pivot
(superior radioulnar)

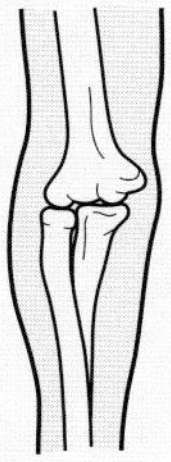

ball and socket (hip)

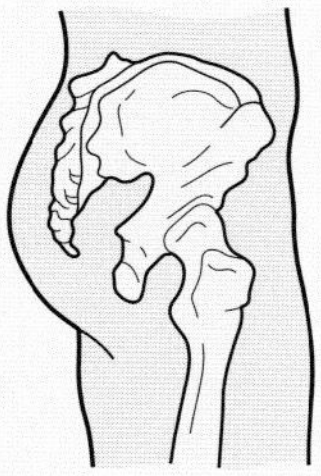

condyloid (metacarpophalangeal)

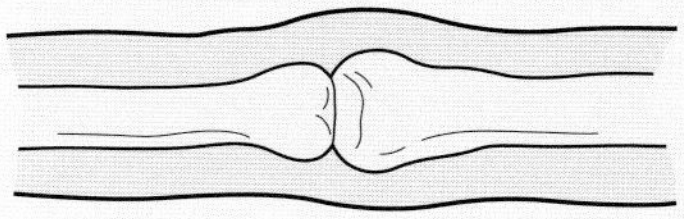

ellipsoid (radiocarpal)

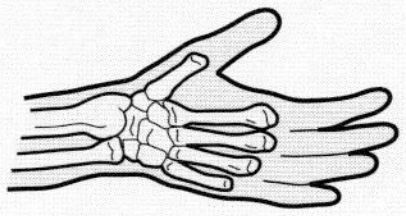

Synovial joints

The synovial joints are the ones we are most concerned with when using stretching exercises. They move freely and contain a variety of joint structures. A typical synovial joint consists of two bone-ends covered by articular cartilage (*see* fig 2.2). The joint is surrounded by a fibrous joint capsule. Certain portions of the capsule are thickened to form supporting ligaments. The capsule is lined with a thin synovial membrane that secretes a lubricating liquid called *synovial fluid*. Structures inside the joint or within the capsule are known as *intracapsular*. Structures associated with the joint but found outside the capsule are called *extracapsular*. These include small balloon-like pads or *bursae* which stop structures rubbing over each other, and small 'fat pads' that fill the gaps between tissues.

Muscles control the joint, and those passing close to the bones may attach some fibres to the joint structures. For example, the popliteus muscle of the knee also attaches to the medial knee ligament and medial knee meniscus.

There are seven main types of synovial joints (*see* table 2.1).

- The **plane** joint has relatively flat surfaces and permits gliding or twisting of one bone against the other. The intertarsal joints of the foot are examples of plane joints.
- The **saddle** joint has one convex surface and one concave surface arranged at right angles to each other, as with a horse rider sitting in a saddle. The major movements occur in two planes, with a slight amount of combined movement occurring in a third plane. An example is the carpometacarpal (CMC) joint of the thumb.
- The **hinge** joint allows movement in one axis only, and a strong joint is formed with tight ligaments. An example is the elbow joint (humeroulnar), formed between the humerus and ulna.

- The **pivot** joint allows a rotation movement about one axis only. One piece of bone rotates in a ring formed by the other bone and ligament tissue. An example is the joint formed between the radius and the ulna in the elbow (superior radioulnar).
- The **ball and socket** joint allows movement in all three planes, examples being the hip and shoulder joints. A ball-shaped surface of one bone articulates with a cup-shaped surface of the other.
- The **condyloid** joint is similar to the ball and socket, but allows movement in only two planes. The metacarpophalangeal (MCP) joints of the fingers are examples.
- The **ellipsoid** joint is again a modification of the ball and socket. The convex surface of one bone is oval in shape, while the concave surface of the opposing bone is elliptical. The radio-carpal joint in the wrist is an example here.

> **Key point**: Consider the type of joint being strength training than to stretching. However, moved during a stretching exercise. Does it actually because stretching is primarily affecting muscle, it is permit the movement you are trying to develop?

Joint structures

Individual differences in joint structures

Although each person has the same joint types, there is tremendous variation in the general structure and function of joints between two individuals.

The shapes of the bones will vary. This can be due to hereditary influences, physical training or injury. Some people are naturally more, or less, flexible because of the shapes of their bones.

Those who have exercised regularly since an early age will be considerably different from

Figure 2.2 Typical synovial joint structure

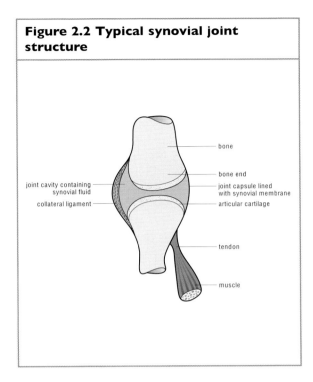

- bone
- bone end
- joint capsule lined with synovial membrane
- articular cartilage
- joint cavity containing synovial fluid
- collateral ligament
- tendon
- muscle

Table 2.2	Tissue Types
Tissue	**Function**
Epithelial	Tightly packed cells which form coverings and make up skin and outer coating of organs
Connective	Loose cells in fluid base which modify to form joint structures
Muscular	Contracts muscles
Nervous	Conducts electrical impulses

Connective tissue and the formation of joint structures

The tissues of the body are of four basic types (*see* table 2.2). *Epithelial* tissue consists of densely packed cells that form coverings, and makes up skin and the outer coating of organs. Connective tissue (described below) consists of loosely arranged cells. *Muscular* tissue has the ability to contract, and nervous tissue to conduct electrical impulses.

Connective tissue is composed of cells floating within a fluid known as an *extracellular matrix*. The composition of the cells and matrix determines the type and function of the particular connective tissue described. The cells have many functions including creating and maintaining the fluid matrix and ultimately breaking it down. Three types of fibres are found within the matrix. *Collagen* fibres are the most abundant and are so profuse that they may form one third of the total body-weight. The collagen fibres have a rope-like appearance and are strong but non-elastic. The second type of fibre found is *elastin.* This resembles a coiled spring and has great elastic capacities. The elastin fibres crisscross each other to form a net, similar to the springs in a bed mattress. The third type of fibre is *reticular* fibre. Reticular fibres are really a type of collagen, and are very fine fibres that branch to form a meshwork.

inactive individuals. For example, girls who have spent many years practising ballet as children will tend to be more flexible around the hips for the rest of their lives.

Injury and disease will also affect the range of motion possible at a joint. Older athletes who have varying amounts of arthritis will show reduced movement in specific patterns. For example, lateral rotation of the shoulder and hip tends to be very limited. Where an injury has occurred early in life, the growth plate in a bone may have been affected. A severe fall from a bicycle or horse can often dislodge a bony growth plate and alter the formation of the final mature bone.

The structural differences at a joint must be appreciated when comparing ranges of movement between individuals. Even with the same amount of training, two people may never gain the same amount of movement at a joint.

The basic design of connective tissue is modified to form the various joint structures described below.

Types of joint structures

Articular cartilage

The ends of the bones forming a joint are covered by articular (hyaline) cartilage, a modified connective tissue. The cartilage matrix contains specialised cells known as *chondrocytes*, which maintain its integrity. It also contains both collagen and elastin fibres in varying proportions together with proteoglycan, a protein that acts as a sponge to trap water, giving cartilage an exceptionally high (70–80 per cent) water content. Cartilage has no blood vessels or nerves, relying instead for its nutrition on the synovial fluid. Substances move into and out of the cartilage by diffusion from the synovial fluid, a process heavily reliant on regular movement to cause alterations in pressure within the fluid. As the cartilage is compressed intermittently with movement, for example walking or running, nutrients are pumped into and out of the cartilage. With continuous loading, such as occurs in prolonged standing, the cartilage is compressed further and further without allowing more fluid to be taken up. This continual compression without release can reduce the cartilage depth by as much as 40 per cent.

The area of cartilage next to the bone (the sub-chondral region) is firmly attached to the bone and will resist shearing stresses. The main body of the cartilage contains fibres that will resist tension stresses, while the fluid within the cartilage gel resists compression stresses. The fibres are elastic, and the gel will gradually flow away from any compressing force. It is the combination of these two reactions that gives cartilage a viscoelastic property.

The joint capsule

The joint capsule is composed of two parts. The outer portion (*stratum fibrosum*) is tough and fibrous, and is thickened in certain areas to form ligaments. The inner portion of the capsule (*stratum synoviale*) is loose and contains many blood vessels. This region blends with the synovial membrane of the joint.

The capsule is attached to the bones around the edge of the joint, and at the line of attachments many small blood vessels are seen. The capsule has a rich supply of nerve fibres responsible for the 'joint sense' (proprioception) used in balance and reflex actions. The capsule is particularly important after injury. Following joint sprains, the joint will swell, and the accumulation of fluid will stretch the capsule causing tightness and pain. After injury, the capsule can thicken and further limit the joint movement, requiring specialist physiotherapy techniques and regular stretching exercises to regain the lost movement.

Synovial membrane

The synovial membrane lines the joint capsule and consists of two distinct layers. The inner layer secretes the synovial fluid, while the outer layer is a loose, highly vascular structure consisting of collagen fibres and fat cells. This outer layer merges with the membrane covering the bones, the *periosteum*.

The blood vessels of the joint divide into three branches: one travelling to the epiphysis at the end of the bone; the second to the joint capsule; and the third to the synovial membrane itself. The blood vessels contained in the synovial membrane can exchange fluid and nutrient molecules with the synovial fluid. The synovial membrane has a series of folds in it and, as the joint moves, it will unfold like a fan to allow movement (rather than simply stretching). The folds of the synovial membrane have extensive lubrication to virtually eliminate friction.

Ligaments

Many ligaments are simply parts of the joint capsule that have thickened to resist particular stresses on the joints. They are made of connective tissue fibres, and attach to the bones of the joint. The ligament fibres are arranged along the lines of stress imposed on the joint. As a joint moves, the ligaments will stretch, initially pulling the fibres straight and then stretching them. Exercise will regularly lengthen the ligaments and strengthen them, but stretching exercises that overstress the ligaments should be avoided. The ligaments support the joint, and, if overstretched, can leave the joint too flexible, causing it to be insecure and open to injury. Following a ligament injury, it is particularly important to keep the joint moving gently, so that the newly healing ligament fibres will again align themselves correctly, rather than in a haphazard fashion.

Ligaments at the side of the joint (collateral ligaments) resist stresses which would tend to open the joint sideways. Other ligaments are positioned to protect the joint in its most vulnerable movements. For example, in the knee the cruciate ligaments prevent the thighbone (femur) from sliding forwards and backwards on the shinbone (tibia), and in the shoulder the glenohumeral ligament prevents the ball of the shoulder (head of humerus) from moving too far forwards in its socket (glenoid) and dislocating.

Consideration must be given to ligaments when stretching at all times. Stretches that are excessive or brutal in their application may actually damage the ligamentous support of a joint and cause severe injury.

Muscle–tendon unit

The muscles are attached to the bones via a tendon. This is an inelastic collagen structure that simply transmits the force created by the muscle to the bone in order to move it. The tendon is able to transmit the force to a small area,

keeping the bulk of the muscle away from the joint. Some tendons, such as those of the finger muscles, are very long, allowing the muscles to be positioned in the forearm, well away from the finger joint where the muscle force is applied. Other tendons, such as that of the deltoid muscle of the shoulder, are right next to the muscle itself.

The thick, central part of the muscle is called the muscle belly, and it is this part that bulges as the muscle contracts. The muscle then tapers down towards the tendon and this area between the muscle and tendon is called the musculotendinous junction. The tendon then inserts into the bone via the teno-osseous junction.

Fascia

Muscle is contained within a framework of connective tissue called *fascia*. The fascia forms compartments (*see* chapter 3) that contain the contractile fibres of the muscle itself. If you were to take a piece of muscle and dry it by removing all the water, the dry powder that would remain represents the building blocks of the muscle. Although most of us think of muscles as giving strength and contracting to lift weights, for example, in actual fact the dry weight of the contractile proteins of a muscle is about equal to the dry weight of the non-contractile material. In other words, there is as much non-contractile fascia within a muscle are there is contractile tissue!

So what does all this fascia do? In addition to providing the framework that holds the muscle together, fascia can actually create force, not through contraction but through elastic recoil. As you stretch a muscle, it will spring back or recoil partly because of the elasticity of fascia. In addition, some muscles attach to bones not via tendons, but by tendinous sheets of fascia each called an *aponeurosis*. In this case, the fascia transmits some of the force created by the muscle. Finally, between each major muscle, the fascia is thickened into a structure called the *intermuscular septum*. This is the thick white 'marbling' that you see in meat when you cut it across.

Although muscles are each separate structures, their fascias are joined together into a tough fibrous network. In some areas, these fascias become specialised and have a specific name attributed to them. In the back, for example, there is the thoroco-lumbar fascia (TLF), and on the outside of the thigh there is the iliotibial band (ITB). The importance of fascia from the point of view of stretching is that a stretch will often affect several muscles at once, all of which are linked by fascial pathways or 'tracts'. To describe the effect of movements on both the muscle and fascia at the same time, we use the term *myofascia*, meaning the contractile muscle fibres and the fascial framework surrounding it.

> **Key point**: When designing stretching exercises for individual muscles, consider that the muscles may actually be linked together in myofascial tracts.

Lubrication of joint cartilage

The articular cartilage has no blood supply. As we have seen, it relies largely for its nutrition on materials being passed from the synovial fluid. Movement will flush fresh fluid over the cartilage surface, and alterations in pressure will press nutrients into the cartilage. If the joint does not move properly, for example following injury, nutrient material may not be pressed into the cartilage, and that area may degenerate, giving osteoarthritis.

The synovial fluid provides a lubricating mechanism that cuts down the amount of friction the joint is subjected to. As the two bony surfaces move over each other, the small synovial fluid molecules act as tiny ball-bearings preventing the opposing cartilage surfaces from rubbing away. Some of the fluid is absorbed into the cartilage almost like water in a sponge. As pressure is exerted on the joint, for example when standing or walking, the fluid is squeezed out of the cartilage to form a fluid film that separates the cartilage surfaces and again prevents them rubbing.

It is often said (usually by inactive individuals) that exercise causes arthritis. This is far from the case. Movement will actually keep the joint cartilage healthy and is essential for the general health of the joint. However, if an injury occurs and an athlete tries to 'train through the pain', the biomechanics of the joint will be altered and changes may occur in the joint cartilage, ultimately leading to the development of arthritis. In addition, a balance must be kept between the strength of muscles supporting a joint and the flexibility of the joint structures. If a person becomes too flexible, the joint will not be secure. Similarly, if a person has too little flexibility, their joints will be stiff. Either case will alter the normal biomechanics of a joint and could give problems later in life.

> **Key point**: Joint cartilage needs regular movement to give it nutrition and keep it healthy.

Joint mechanics

Physiological and accessory movements

Two major types of movement are possible at any joint. First, there are the normal actions that an athlete controls, such as flexion and extension. These are known as *physiological* movements. But there are also *accessory* movements, which cannot be produced directly but occur automatically as a joint moves, giving 'joint play'. For example, as the knee bends and straightens, the

Figure 2.3 Accessory movements in a joint

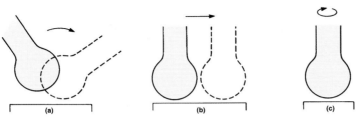

(a)   (b)   (c)

femur and tibia will also glide and roll on each other. The bending and straightening (flexion and extension) are the physiological movements, while the gliding and rolling are the accessory movements. Three distinct types of accessory movements occur, known as *roll, slide* and *spin.*

Roll is similar to a car tyre rolling over the road surface. At any point, the same areas on the tyre will be in contact with the same areas on the road surface (*see* fig 2.3(a)). If slide occurs, a single point on one surface will be in contact with a number of other points on the opposing surface, as when a car tyre skids (*see* fig 2.3(b)). Spin occurs when both points on the two opposing surfaces are in contact, and pure rotation occurs as with a 'spinning top' (*see* fig 2.3(c)).

Accessory movements become important to general flexibility after injury. If a joint is stiff, stretching it will regain the physiological movements but may not bring back the accessory movements. This can leave the joint feeling awkward and open to injury. For this reason, it is always wise to see a physiotherapist after a sports injury to have the joint movement properly assessed.

Close and loose pack

The two opposing surfaces of a joint do not fit together exactly – they are said to be *non-congruent.* However, with the joint in one particular position its surfaces will come as close together as they are able, and this is known as 'close pack'. In this position the joint capsule and ligaments twist and pull the joint surfaces tightly together. The joint space is at a minimum, the concave surface of one bone fits closely on to the convex shape of the other, and no further movement is possible. In the close-pack position, stress will be taken on the bones in a fall because the ligaments in a joint are fully tightened and unable to 'give' any more. A fracture is often the result.

The loose-pack position is exactly the opposite. As the joint surfaces are released from their close-pack position, elastic recoil of the soft tissues surrounding the joint enables its surfaces to move apart, maximizing the joint space. The joint will be less secure in this position and more movement will be possible. Should the athlete fall with the joint in a loose-pack position, the joint will often move too much, and ligament injury can result.

Key point: A loose-pack position, where the joint structures are relaxed and the joint surfaces have moved apart, will facilitate free movement.

Summary

- There are over 200 bones in the body, each made from calcium, phosphorous and proteins.

- Most bones begin life as cartilage and harden through a process of ossification.
- Synovial joints are surrounded by a capsule strengthened by ligaments.
- The joint contains synovial fluid, and the bone ends are covered by cartilage.
- Joints need regular movement to stay healthy.

- Joints have two types of movement: physiological and accessory.
- Physiological movements consist of bending, straightening and twisting, while accessory movements give the joint its healthy spring.
- In the close-pack position a joint is locked, whereas in the loose-pack position it moves freely.

MUSCLE ACTION

How muscles work

Muscle contraction itself is more important to vital that we have some understanding of the general principles underlying muscle actions.

Structure of a muscle

Muscle membranes

If we take a small piece of muscle tissue and magnify it many times (*see* fig 3.1(a)), we can see that it is made up of many long muscle fibres. Each individual muscle fibre is surrounded by a thin membrane (*endomysium*), and in turn the fibres are grouped together in bundles covered by the *perimysium*. Finally, the whole muscle structure is encased in a sheath, the *epimysium*.

The muscle membranes stretch the whole length of the muscle from tendon to tendon, intimately linking the contractile and inert portions of the muscle. The whole structure is often referred to as the 'musculo-tendinous unit'. The muscle membranes are part of the fascia (see Chapter 13). This not only encases the muscles, but actually spreads across and between muscle groups linking them together in fascial pathways.

The combination of fibre contraction and elastic recoil of the muscle membranes is important for the development of 'elastic strength' (*see* page 34). Therefore, stretches that target myofascial pathways are important for speed and power sports involving the whole body, such as martial arts and dance.

> **Key point**: Muscle membranes link several muscles together and are important in the development of 'elastic strength'. They should be considered when stretching for power sports in particular.

Muscle microstructure

A further membrane, the *sarcolemma*, surrounds the individual muscle cells. The sarcolemma is important because it is electrically conductive; it has within it *sarcoplasm*, a fluid containing fuel stores (*glycogen*) and enzymes important to muscle contraction. Within the sarcoplasm is an intricate membrane, the *sarcoplasmic reticulum*. This membrane contains transverse tubules, each of which end on the muscle cell surface as a lateral sac.

Looking closely at each fibre, we see alternating light and dark bands, corresponding to different muscle proteins. The light area is composed of a thin filament called *actin*, while the dark area consists of a thicker filament called *myosin*. The two sets of filaments fit together like the fingers on two opposing hands, one set of actin–myosin fibres being called a *sarcomere*. The thick myosin filament has projections or 'crossbridges' coming from it much like the oars of a boat. The thin actin filament has a long *tropomyosin* filament wound around it and a globular *troponin* molecule is positioned over this area. At rest the tropomyosin prevents (inhibits) actin and myosin from binding.

Figure 3.1(a) Structure of a muscle – contractile mechanism: (a) whole muscle and a group of muscle fibres; (b) a myofibril; (c) a sarcomere; (d) thick and thin filaments

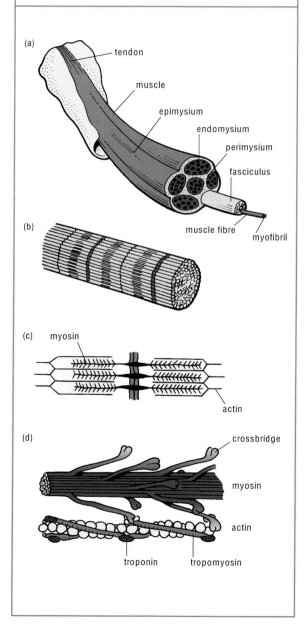

How do muscles contract?

Contraction of the muscle occurs when the muscle filaments move towards each other, and a whole sequence of events is required for this to take place. When we want a muscle to contract, a nervous impulse is sent from the brain. This impulse travels down the spinal cord and along a peripheral nerve to the muscle, where it causes changes on the surface of the muscle fibre. At the point where the nerve touches the muscle, a chemical (*acetylcholine*) is released, which causes an electrical impulse to spread across the surface of the sarcolemma. As a result, calcium is released from the lateral sacs and passes down the transverse tubule to bind with the troponin molecule (*see* fig 3.1(b)). This reaction causes the spiral trompomyosin to move deeper into the groove of the actin filament removing the inhibition. Once the inhibition has been removed, contraction will occur spontaneously, and the muscle filaments pull closer together, causing them to slide over each other and shorten the muscle.

The whole muscle contraction process uses energy, and rest is needed to recharge the structures involved. Calcium has to be moved out of the transverse tubule of the muscle and back into

Figure 3.1(b) Structure of a muscle – transverse tubule system

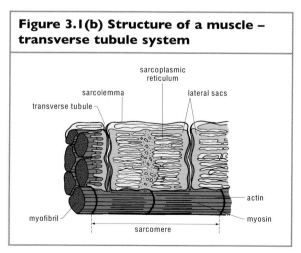

the lateral sacs. The filaments must then return to their original relaxed positions.

What affects muscle strength?

The amount of overlap that can occur between the sliding filaments of the muscle will determine its *contractile strength*, and the relationship between muscle length and tension development is called the length–tension relationship (*see* fig 3.2). When the muscle is shortened, the filaments are overlapped already and have little additional movement available to them. In the shortened position (inner range), therefore, the muscle is comparatively 'weak'. In the lengthened position (outer range), the filaments have pulled apart and the actin and myosin elements are disengaged. Again the muscle is relatively 'weak' – it can produce little active force through contraction – however, because the muscle is now stretched, it is able to produce some force through elastic recoil, known as elastic strength. Therefore, the force in the outer range is mostly created passively through recoil, rather than actively through contraction.

It is only in mid-range, when the muscle filaments are engaged but not overlapping, that maximal active force can be developed. Mid-range is the range that we use in our normal day-to-day activities, so functionally it is appropriate that this should be the strongest point in the available movement.

> **Key point**: Contractile strength results from muscle contraction, while elastic strength comes from muscle recoil as a result of elasticity in the stretched muscle and reflex mechanisms.

Muscle reflexes

Three muscle reflexes are important when using flexibility training: the *stretch reflex*; *autogenic inhibition* (also known as the reverse stretch reflex); and *reciprocal innervation*.

Stretch reflex

The *stretch reflex* is important both for postural control and muscle tone. It relies on information coming from special receptors called *muscle spindles* (*see* fig 3.3(a)). The muscle spindle is a cigar-shaped structure attached alongside

---

Figure 3.2 Length–tension relationship of a muscle

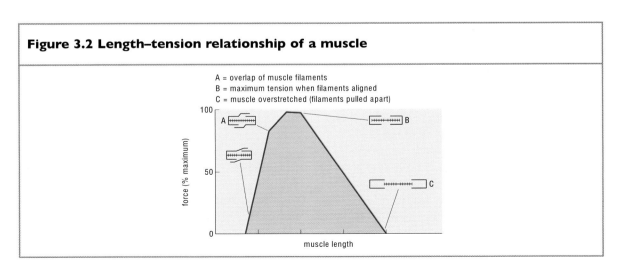

A = overlap of muscle filaments
B = maximum tension when filaments aligned
C = muscle overstretched (filaments pulled apart)

Figure 3.3(a) Muscle receptors

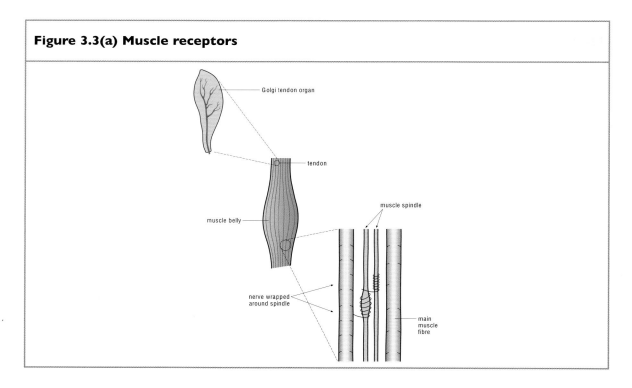

Golgi tendon organ

tendon

muscle spindle

muscle belly

nerve wrapped around spindle

main muscle fibre

the main muscle fibres. When the muscle is stretched, so is the muscle spindle. The stretch of the spindle is detected by nerves, and a reflex occurs that causes the muscle to contract and shorten the spindle once more.

The stretch reflex reacts to change in both the length of the muscle and in the velocity of its movement. Change in length is important for postural or *tonic* control, while change in velocity is important for movement or *phasic* control. The classic example of the stretch reflex acting for phasic control is the knee jerk, or patellar reflex. Here, the patella tendon is stretched rapidly by being hit with a small rubber hammer. This rapid stretch is picked up by the muscle spindles in the quadriceps and causes nerve impulses to be sent to the spinal cord. Impulses return from the cord to the quadriceps causing them to contract, and the knee straightens quickly giving a small 'kick'.

The stretch reflex is also essential for the maintenance of normal standing posture through tonic control. When we stand up we continually sway forwards and backwards. As we start to fall forwards, there is a pull on our calf muscles, changing their length and causing a stretch reflex. The calf muscles then contract a split second later to pull us back to the upright position again.

The reflex occurs in three parts (*see* fig 3.3(b)). The first response is a short latency contraction (M1), which results from activation of the spinal reflex circuit itself. The second response is a long latency contraction (M2), which involves the lower centres of the brain. The third response, (M3), occurs occasionally and is again a result of brain activity rather than the spinal cord. Voluntary contractions can occur within 170 ms of the detection of a movement, but the stretch reflex occurs much faster. M1 occurs within 30 ms and M2 within 50 to 60 ms. The stretch reflex

Figure 3.3(b) Muscle activity during the stretch reflex

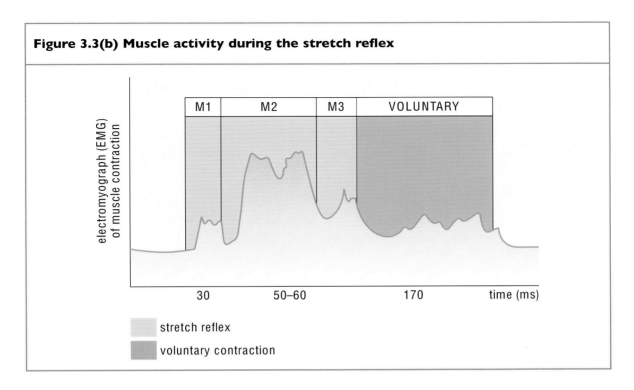

therefore causes muscle contraction in response to an unexpected stretch some 140 ms (nearly one-fifth of a second) before voluntary muscle contraction.

The result is that the stretch initiates a contraction of the same muscle that limits the stretch itself, creating a negative feedback system sometimes referred to as a *resistance reflex*. The reflex is protective, tending to stabilise a joint, and relies on a continuous barrage of nerve impulses coming from the joint itself. This process is known as 'joint sense' or *proprioception*.

After injury, these nerve impulses can be lessened (proprioception is impaired) tending to make a joint less stable. Therefore, an essential part of sports rehabilitation is the use of training to increase the number of nerve impulses being fed to a joint. This is achieved by performing a large variety of movements, especially those which tax balance skills, as these will feed more and more nerve impulses into the joint. This type of training, known as proprioceptive exercise, will help to restore the stability of a joint by improving the 'reaction time' of the muscles supporting it. In this way the stretch reflex is restored to its correct level of action and it is able once more to support the joint.

Key point: Proprioception is often impaired following injury, and needs to be retrained using special exercises based on balance and stability.

Autogenic inhibition

Another receptor, the *golgi tendon organ* (GTO), is situated in the muscle tendon (see fig 3.3(a)). This receptor measures tension. When a muscle contracts, it shortens, so a stretch reflex will not occur. However, the GTO will register

31

the increasing tension in the muscle tendon and will then cause a reflex relaxation of the muscle, a process known as *autogenic inhibition.* This is the reverse situation to the stretch reflex and has a protective function, preventing the muscle from contracting so hard that it pulls its attachment off the bone. The two reflexes do not occur at the same time, because the threshold of the GTO is set far higher than that of the muscle spindle. In normal everyday movement, tension in the muscle is not high enough to cause autogenic inhibition.

Both stretch and autogenic inhibition reflexes have important implications for stretching exercises. Stretching that involves short jerking movements will tighten the muscle through the stretch reflex, while sustained stretching (over about 30 seconds) will allow the muscle to relax. Relaxation occurs because the stretch reflex becomes desensitised, and, if the muscle tension is high enough, autogenic inhibition follows through stimulation of the GTO. The autogenic inhibition in this case overrides the stretch reflex.

Reciprocal innervation

A further reflex is called *reciprocal innervation.* This occurs when the antagonist muscle relaxes to allow the prime mover to create a movement. For example, when the biceps muscle contracts to bend the elbow, the triceps will relax through reciprocal innervation to allow the movement to occur. This reflex can be used to obtain further relaxation in a muscle just prior to stretching.

> **Key point**: The stretch reflex increases muscle tone in response to muscle stretch, autogenic inhibition reduces tone when tension detected in a tendon is too great and reciprocal innervation relaxes a muscle when its neighbour contracts.

Elastic and contractile properties of muscle

Muscle has three properties: contractibility, elasticity and extensibility.

Contractibility

The contractile nature of muscle results from the movement of the sliding filaments within the muscle fibre.

Isometric

When the actin and myosin filaments come together, force is generated and the muscle will shorten. If the muscle filaments shorten, but the external length of the muscle remains the same, the muscle tenses but the joint on which the muscle works will not move. This is an *isometric* or static muscle contraction. An example is holding an object in the hand with the elbow bent to 90°.

Concentric

When the muscle filaments shorten and pull the attachments of the muscle closer to each other, causing movement at the joint, the muscle contraction is then *concentric.* In our example above, instead of the arm being held still, the elbow joint flexes. A concentric action tends to accelerate a limb. The movement begins slowly and gets faster.

Eccentric

Once the elbow has been flexed, and the muscle filaments shortened, lowering the weight again involves the muscle filaments slowly paying out to control the joint as it extends. This is an *eccentric* action. This type of action is used to slow the body down and control movements such as sitting down into a chair or coming downstairs. Each time, the muscle filaments are sliding apart and the muscle is lengthening.

Key point: In isometric contraction the joint does not move; concentric contraction causes acceleration; and eccentric contraction causes deceleration.

Elasticity

Individual muscle fibres are grouped together in bundles (*see* page 28) and each fibre is surrounded by a connective tissue sheath (the endomysium). The bundles themselves are again aligned in groups and surrounded by another sheath (the epimysium). The muscle sheaths cannot contract, but they will stretch, and they have important elastic properties. These elements of the muscle are known as the *parallel elastic components* because they are aligned parallel to the muscle fibres. The tendons at the end of the muscle are also non-contractile, but again they show elastic properties. These are the *series elastic components*, so called because they are positioned before and after the fibres.

We know that there is a linear relationship between load and elasticity from the load–deformation curve (*see* page 10). As we load a muscle it will stretch proportionally, and, as the stretch ceases and the muscle springs back, energy is released.

Extensibility

If the stretch is applied slowly and released slowly, so that the muscle remains relaxed (non-contractile), the force produced by the muscle is purely passive. This is important in posture especially. As we bend forwards to touch our toes, the back muscles (erector spinae) are lengthening eccentrically to lower the trunk. However, these same muscles are also being placed on stretch. When we begin to come back up from the forward bend position, initially there is no muscle contraction. We begin our upward movement purely through elastic recoil

Figure 3.3(c) Flexion–relaxation response: (a) body is lowered by eccentric activity of the back muscles; (b) at full flexion the back muscles are fully stretched; (c) recoil of the stretched muscles begins the upward trunk movement – no muscle contraction is required initially

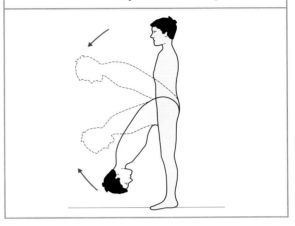

of the back muscles, a process known as the *flexion–relaxation response* (*see* fig 3.3(c)). This mechanism is simply a way of conserving muscle energy, but it does illustrate the importance of maintaining healthy elasticity within a muscle. For example, if a person suffers from chronic low back pain, the flexion–relaxation response no longer occurs because the back muscles are continuously in spasm and are unable to relax and stretch. The result is that the muscles have a poor blood flow (because blood no longer pumps through the muscle as it contracts and relaxes) and acids build up in the muscles causing pain.

As stretches become more rapid, the force produced is a combination of both elastic and contractile properties. When we lengthen a muscle its filaments move apart, ready to contract once more, and the elastic elements of the muscle are stretched. If this stretch is applied

Figure 3.4 Developing elastic strength

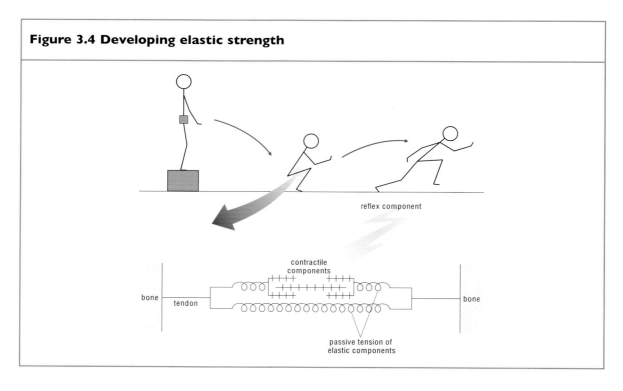

rapidly, a stretch reflex occurs, causing the muscle to tighten and pull against the stretching force. If the muscle contracts immediately afterwards, the contractile force produced will be a summation of contraction, elastic recoil, and reflex mechanisms and will be far greater than if the muscle contracted from rest (*see* fig 3.4). This type of pre-stretching is used to advantage in plyometric training where a series of jumps and bounding movements are used to build up 'elastic strength'.

> **Key point**: Elastic strength comes from (a) muscle contraction, (b) elastic recoil and (c) reflex contract.

Muscle fibres

Types of muscle fibres

All muscles contain fibres of different types. Red fibres are designed to contract over and over again without fatiguing, and are known as *slow-twitch* fibres. White fibres are called *fast twitch*, and these give short bursts of power. A person's muscles will contain both fibre types, but in different proportions. Those who are good at endurance sports tend to have more slow-twitch fibres in the leg muscles, while those who perform explosive sprints have more fast-twitch fibres (*see* fig 3.5).

Arrangement of muscle fibres

No matter which type is present, each muscle fibre is only able to shorten and reduce its length by half. Although the same amount of shortening occurs with each fibre, altering the arrangement of these fibres within a muscle will affect muscle function. Two different arrangements are found, one for short powerful muscles and the other for long flexible ones.

Figure 3.5 Distribution of fibre types

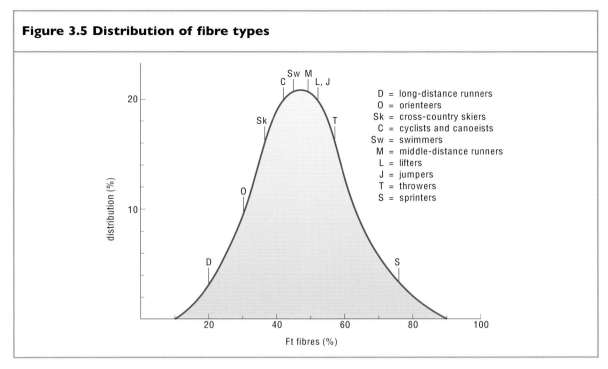

D = long-distance runners
O = orienteers
Sk = cross-country skiers
C = cyclists and canoeists
Sw = swimmers
M = middle-distance runners
L = lifters
J = jumpers
T = throwers
S = sprinters

The short powerful type is like the deltoid muscle of the shoulder. Here, the fibres are arranged side by side, inserting into a central tendon like the barbs on a feather. There are many of them so the muscle is very powerful. However, the fibres are short so the muscle cannot move very far and is therefore comparatively inflexible. This type of arrangement is called *pennate* (*see* fig 3.6(a)).

Long slender muscles like the hamstrings on the back of the leg have their fibres arranged parallel to each other, attaching to tendons at each end (*see* fig 3.6(b)). This type of muscle is called *fusiform*. There are fewer fibres, so the muscle is less powerful. However, the muscle will still shorten by half, and, as this type of muscle is much longer, the movement it produces will be of a greater range. When choosing stretching exercises it is important to be aware of the underlying muscle structure to devise more effective programmes.

If we are throwing an object or hitting a ball we often need to develop the maximal amount of force possible. The amount of force will be dependent on our underlying strength, but also on the flexibility of a muscle and on the range of

Figure 3.6 Arrangement of muscle fibres: (a) shorter fibres of pennate muscle; (b) longer fibres of parallel muscles

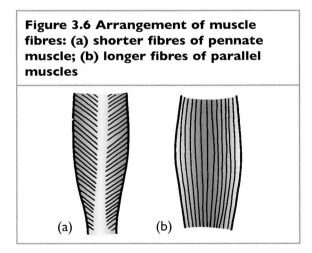

(a)   (b)

Table 3.1	Group action of muscles (example: elbow flexion)			
Prime mover (agonist)	Secondary (assistant) mover	Antagonist	Stabilisor (fixator)	Neutraliser
Creates primary movement (biceps)	Assists prime mover (brachialis)	If contracted, would oppose prime mover (triceps)	Stabilises or fixes bone origin of prime mover (shoulder muscles)	Removes unwanted action of prime mover (pronators)

motion through which a limb is taken. This is because when we are able to use a greater range of motion, we have more time to allow the speed of an object to build up. Take as an example the javelin throw. If an athlete has very stiff shoulders, he or she will not be able to take the javelin very far back. An athlete with good flexibility around the shoulders will be able to develop greater force by accelerating the javelin for a longer period.

> Key point: Pennate muscles, being short and stocky, are built for power. Fusiform muscles are long and slender, producing high levels of mobility.

Group action of muscles

A muscle can only pull, it cannot decide which action to perform. We produce an infinite variety of actions with a finite number of muscles by combining the various actions in different ways. This co-ordinated action of the various muscles working on a body-part is called the *group action of muscles* (*see* table 3.1).

Prime mover (agonist)

When a muscle pulls to create a movement it is said to be acting as a *prime mover* or *agonist*. Most muscles can take on this function, depending on the action required and the site of the

muscle. Other muscles may be able to help with the action, but are less effective than the prime mover. The muscles that help are called *secondary* or *assistant movers*. If we take elbow flexion as an example, both biceps and brachialis can flex the elbow. In most circumstances, the biceps is more effective and so acts as the prime mover, with the brachialis as the secondary mover.

Antagonist

The muscle that would oppose the prime mover if it is contracted is known as the *antagonist*. If we bend the arm, the biceps will act as the prime mover to create the power necessary to carry out the movement. To allow the movement to occur, however, the opposite muscle – in this case the triceps – must relax and in so doing acts as an antagonist (*see* fig 3.7).

Stabiliser (fixator)

Muscles do not simply create movements; they are also able to stabilise parts of the body or prevent unwanted actions by acting as *stabilisers* or *fixators*. In this case, the muscle will contract to steady or support the bone on to which the prime mover attaches. Take as an example the sit-up exercise. The abdominal muscles attach from the rib-cage to the pelvis, so when they contract they will move both body areas, tending to posteriorly tilt the pelvis and pull the rib-cage down. To allow the abdominals to contract more

Figure 3.7 Group action of muscles: (a) prime mover/antagonist; (b) fixator; (c) neutraliser

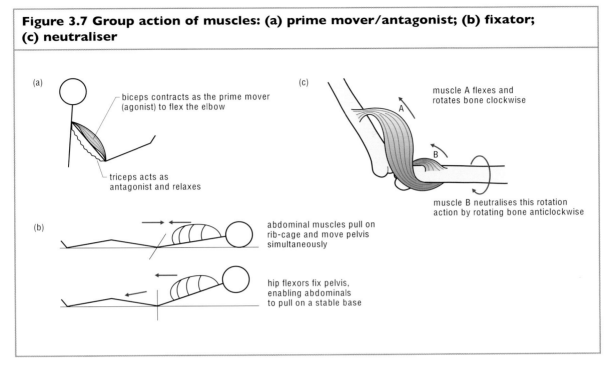

(a)

biceps contracts as the prime mover (agonist) to flex the elbow

triceps acts as antagonist and relaxes

(b)

abdominal muscles pull on rib-cage and move pelvis simultaneously

hip flexors fix pelvis, enabling abdominals to pull on a stable base

(c)

muscle A flexes and rotates bone clockwise

A

B

muscle B neutralises this rotation action by rotating bone anticlockwise

effectively, we need to fix one body area to provide a firm base for the muscles to pull on. This occurs by the hip flexor muscles acting as fixators to stop the pelvis from tilting as the abdominals contract. In the case of elbow flexion, mentioned above, because the biceps attach to the shoulder girdle, these bones must be stabilised to stop them sliding on the rib-cage as the biceps contracts.

Neutraliser

Many muscles can perform more than one movement. In the case of the biceps, for example, as well as flexing the elbow the muscle can also twist the forearm upwards (*supination*). If we want the biceps to perform just one action, bending the arm but not twisting it, other muscles must contract to stop the biceps from twisting the forearm. These muscles, which eliminate unwanted actions, are acting as *neutralisers*. As we saw

above, the biceps muscle cannot decide which action to perform and which not to perform. Again it must be emphasised that a muscle can only pull: if we want to alter the action it will produce, we must bring other muscles into play as neutralisers.

Two-joint muscles

Some muscles cross over two joints, and are said to be *biarticular*. The hamstrings, for example, attach from the seat bone (ischial tuberosity) to the top of the tibia. Because they cross both the hip and knee joints they are capable of creating, or limiting, movement at both joints. Other biarticular muscles include the rectus femoris and gastrocnemius in the lower limbs, and the biceps and triceps in the upper limbs. Biarticular muscles have a number of important biomechanical features.

Passive insufficiency

First, because they pass over two joints, they cannot shorten enough to allow full movement at both joints simultaneously. For example, with the knee bent and the hamstrings relaxed at the knee, the hip can flex maximally enabling the knee to be pulled right up on to the chest (*see* fig 3.8). However, with the knee straight, and the lower portion of the hamstrings stretched, hip flexion is more limited. This limitation of movement at both joints is called *passive insufficiency*.

Active insufficiency

If you stand up and flex your hip, you will be able to bend your knee actively to touch your buttock with your heel. If you pull your hip into extension first, however, and try the same movement, you will find that you are unable to touch your heel to your buttock. This is because in the first example the upper portion of the hamstrings was lengthened and the lower part shortened. In the second example, the upper and lower parts of the muscle are unable to shorten fully at the same time. This inability to create full movement at both joints simultaneously is called *active insufficiency*.

> **Key point:** A two-joint (biarticular) muscle such as the hamstring or rectus femoris does not permit full movement at both of the joints it spans at the same time.

Concurrent movement

Because biarticular muscles are unable to permit full movement at both joints at the same time, the tension in one muscle will cause tension to build up in its antagonist. For example, if the hamstrings contract and extend the hip, they will stretch the rectus femoris which is acting as an

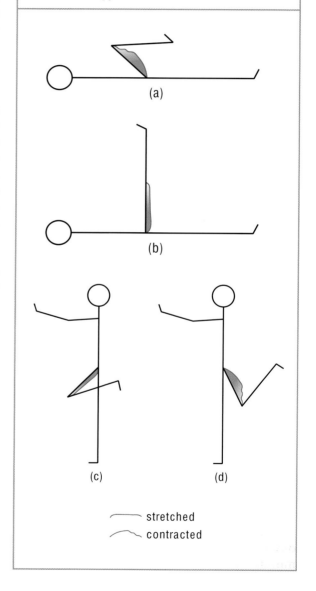

Figure 3.8 Active and passive insufficiency of a muscle: (a) hamstring stretched at the hip but relaxed at the knee; (b) hamstrings stretched over both joints (passive insufficiency); (c) hamstring stretched at the hip and controlled at both joints (active insufficiency)

antagonist. The stretch in the rectus will then tend to pull the knee straight and extend it. When both the hip and knee are extending in this fashion, *concurrent movement* is said to be occurring. If we look at what happens to the muscle, we can see that this type of action actually conserves energy. The hip and knee are both extending, so the hamstrings are shortened at their upper end and lengthened at their lower end. The rectus femoris is shortened at its lower end and lengthened higher up. This action has therefore avoided both active and passive insufficiency, by neither shortening nor stretching both ends of either muscle. It is used in running as we push off from the ground.

Countercurrent movement

In a kicking action the opposite occurs. When the hip is flexed and the knee extended, both the upper and lower portions of the rectus femoris are shortened, while both parts of the hamstrings are lengthened. The rectus therefore rapidly loses tension while the hamstrings rapidly gain tension, an example of *countercurrent movement.*

> Key point: When the two points covered by a biarticular move the in the same direction (e.g. extension–extension), concurrent movement is taking place. When they move in opposite directions (e.g. extension–flexion), the movement is countercurrent.

Muscle imbalance and core stability

Muscles can be broadly categorised into two types, depending on how they function in day-to-day activities (*see* table 3.2). Some muscles, for example gluteals, act as postural

Table 3.2	Muscle imbalance
Stabilising muscles (postural)	**Movement muscles (locomotion)**
Characteristics	Characteristics
Deep	Superficial
Predominantly slow-twitch	Predominantly fast-twitch
Single joint	Two-joint
Reduced activity (inhibited)	Preferential recruitment
Lengthen	Tighten
Light resistance	High resistance and ballistic
Correction	**Correction**
Improve tone and endurance	Stretch the tight muscles

or *stabilising* muscles, while others, for example hamstrings, act as locomotion or *movement* muscles.

Stabilising muscles

Stabilising muscles tend to be placed deeply within the body and act as postural muscles. Examples include the deep abdominals (transversus abdominis) and the deep spinal muscles (multifidus), as well as the gluteals in many situations (*see* table 3.3). These muscles are built for endurance and have many slow-twitch fibres. They contract minimally, but hold the contraction for a long time. Unfortunately, in a person with an inactive lifestyle, or in someone who is active but has poor alignment, the stabilising muscles often have very poor tone and tend to sag. They almost seem to 'give way to gravity'. The tone is poor in these muscles not because they are weak, but because the nerve impulses, which control all muscles, find it difficult to get

Table 3.3	Examples of muscle types
Stabilising muscles	Movement muscles
Deep abdominals	Superficial Abdominals
Gluteals	Hamstrings
Vastus medialis	Rectus femoris
Soleus	Gastrocnemius
Serratus anterior	Pectoralis major
Lower trapezius	Latissimus dorsi

through to the muscle, and we say that the muscle has *poor recruitment.*

The poor recruitment of the muscle occurs because the muscles have been infrequently used, and often because a person has had pain. For example, when a person has knee pain, one of the stabilising muscles of the knee (vastus medialis) will waste, and the same is true of other regions of the body. When we have back pain, our deep abdominals and our deep spinal muscles tend to waste and the nerve impulses to these muscles are reduced. Because the muscles have not been used, we find it difficult to switch them back on – it is a case of 'use it or lose it'.

Key point: Stabilising muscles react to injury by demonstrating poor recruitment. Their tone is low and they take on a sagging appearance.

Movement muscles

Movement muscles, on the other hand, tend to be more superficial, for example the hamstrings on the back of the thigh and rectus femoris on the front. These muscles are very active in sport, being our sprinting and kicking muscles. They work over two joints, in this case the knee and hip, and tend to get very tight and powerful as they are recruited by hard and fast exercise and heavy poundages such as in weight training.

Muscles of this type appear firm to the touch (palpation) and are often painful and hard after long periods of static posture, for example in sitting or standing. They commonly develop focal pain areas known as *trigger points* (TrP) (see also Chapter 14). When touched firmly, the TrP can cause the muscle to contract rapidly and 'jump' or 'flick' painfully. In addition, pressing the TrP can cause pain to travel (refer) along the length of a limb. For example, a TrP in the buttock when pressed firmly can cause pain to spread across the buttock and down into the thigh. TrPs around the scapula commonly give pain across the shoulder and down into the arm. The pain can be intense and burning in nature. There are several methods of releasing a TrP, one of the most effective being stretching, either passively or using the PNF techniques described in chapter 4.

Key point: Movement muscles tend to be tight and may be painful, developing sore focal areas called trigger points.

Correcting the imbalance

Because many forms of training tend to involve harder and faster movements, i.e. 'going for the burn', rather than slow controlled actions, for example yoga and tai chi, we end up with an imbalance of muscle length and tension around a joint. The imbalance leaves us with tight, strong superficial muscles on the one hand and sagging, poorly toned, deeper postural muscles. This gives rise to a number of postural problems and leaves us open to muscle injury through tearing. To correct the imbalance we must do three things: stretch the tight muscles; improve the tone and endurance of the postural muscles by shortening them; and correct any alignment problems which have occurred (*see* fig 3.9).

To begin with we must work for core stability. This involves tightening the abdominal muscles

Figure 3.9 The muscle imbalance process

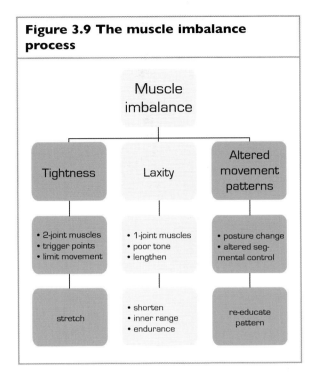

to provide a stable base before we begin stretching. If we fail to do this, as we stretch our alignment may be very poor. In figure 3.10, the subject is trying to stretch the rectus femoris muscle on the front of the thigh by flex-ing the knee and extending the hip at the same time. To do this, the pelvis must remain stable, and must not move. However, in this diagram the subject has been unable to hold the abdom-inal muscles tight enough to stop the pelvis from tilting forwards. They are unable to sta-bilise the lumbo-pelvic region. The stress from this exercise is therefore thrown on to the lower back, potentially causing back injury. For this reason, learning to stabilise the lumbo-pelvic region is essential before lower limb stretching exercises begin. This technique is described on page 73.

Enhancing stability is the start of a longer process of muscle imbalance correction. However, in order to correct the sagging stab-ilising muscles, we must ultimately shorten them, as excessive length rather than poor strength is their major problem. This is achieved by working the muscle only in its inner range rather than in its mid- or outer range. Inner-range work is paralleled with endurance exercise using exercises known as *inner range holding* – liter-ally taking the muscle into its inner range and building up holding time. Instead of adding weight progressively (2 lb, 4 lb, 6 lb etc.), as would be used in weight training, we progress holding time (2 s, 10 s, 30 s etc.).

Figure 3.10 (a) Normal pelvic tilt and lower back alignment; (b) pelvis moves excessively, causing lower back to hollow; leg goes higher, but technique is faulty

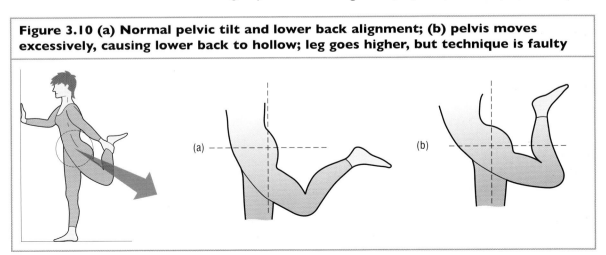

Stretching forms the major part of the management of the shortened movement muscles in the imbalance correction process, and a variety of techniques are covered in the later sections of this book.

Finally, when a person's body has been in a state of imbalance for a long period, the body learns inappropriate *movement patterns* and these must be corrected. Such patterns include bending the back rather than the knees when lifting, hitching the hip when moving the leg sideways and shrugging the shoulder when lifting the arm into abduction. The underlying problem is one of coordination of one part (segment) of the body when moving another, and correction of this process is known as *segmental control.* Modification of general muscle imbalance is out of the realm of this book, and we shall be focusing on stretching the tight movement muscles only. The interested reader is referred to Norris, C.M., (2001), *Abdominal Training: enhancing core stability* (2nd edition), A & C Black, for a user's manual and Norris, C.M., (2000), *Back Stability,* Human Kinetics, for a textbook for therapists.

Summary

- A muscle is made up of actin and myosin filaments, which slide together causing the muscle to mechanisms.
- There are three muscle reflexes relevant to stretching: the stretch reflex, autogenic inhibition and reciprocal innervation.
- Muscle demonstrates contractability (pull), extensibility (stretch) and elasticity (spring).
- Muscles consist of slowtwitch fibres built for endurance and fasttwitch fibres built for power.
- A muscle that creates a movement is a prime mover (agonist); the muscle that relaxes to allow a movement to occur is the antagonist.
- A muscle may also hold a body-part firm (stabiliser) or prevent an unwanted secondary action (neutraliser).
- A biarticular muscle works over two joints.
- Stabilising muscles tend to become lax and sag; movement muscles tighten.
- Muscle imbalance may result in inappropriate movement patterns.

PRINCIPLES OF TRAINING

Warm-up

Before starting any exercise session, it is essential to warm up. There are two main reasons for this: first, warming-up can make sports injuries less likely in certain circumstances; second, the body works more efficiently when warm and sports performance may actually improve. A good warm-up will have physiological, mechanical and psychological effects.

Physiological effects

It takes some time for the body to change from its basic 'tick over' at rest to a point at which it is ready to perform maximally. If vigorous exercise is started immediately from rest, the heartbeat is speeded up with a jolt instead of increasing gradually, and the beats of the heart can become irregular, rather than showing their normal smooth rhythm. These changes affecting the heart can be potentially very serious in the older or less active individual, and especially in those with a history of heart or circulatory problems.

Effects on the heart

In 1973 an important study was conducted which showed the importance of warm-up to the cardio-vascular system (Barnard et al. 1973). Researchers took a group of men with no history of heart problems and made them run vigorously on a treadmill for 10–15 seconds without a warm-up. In 70 per cent of these subjects, abnormal changes were seen on an electro-cardiogram (ECG) machine. These changes, called ischaemia, showed that insufficient blood was getting to the heart muscle, a potentially very dangerous situation. However, when the same subjects ran on the treadmill after performing a warm-up, the ECG changes were greatly reduced, and in many cases the trace was completely normal, demonstrating considerably less strain being imposed on the heart. In addition, blood pressure (BP) was taken when the subjects ran on the treadmill both with and without a warm-up. Average blood pressures of 168 mmHg were taken in those subjects who ran without a warm-up, while for those who did a warm-up the blood pressure averaged 140 mmHg, some 12 per cent lower. Again, these changes demonstrate the importance of a warm-up in reducing the strain placed on the heart by vigorous exercise.

> **Key point**: A warm-up will reduce the strain placed on the heart by vigorous exercise.

Effect on body tissue

A warm-up will allow the body tissues to work more efficiently. Normally, while relaxed, the muscles receive only about 15 per cent of the total blood flow. The rest goes to the body organs such as the brain, liver and intestines. During vigorous exercise, because the muscles need far more fuel to provide energy, their requirement for blood increases and they need 80 per cent of the total blood flow. It takes time to re-route this blood by opening some blood vessels and closing others, and if the muscles are required to perform maximally before the blood flow has changed, they will work inefficiently.

Incidentally, this process of alteration in regional blood flow is the reason why you should not exercise within an hour of eating a heavy meal. After eating, we need the blood to stay in the region of the stomach and intestines to effectively absorb the digested foodstuffs. If we start to exercise during this period, much of the blood will move away from the digestive organs and into the working muscles. The result can be digestive upsets and 'stomach cramps'.

> **Key point**: Changes in regional blood flow mean shunting blood from the body organs to the exercising muscles. Warm-up makes this process smoother and more graduated.

Lactic acid formation

The body can produce energy by two methods: aerobically (with oxygen) and anaerobically (without oxygen). The aerobic method is preferable, because when we work anaerobically we produce a waste product called lactic acid. Unfortunately, we cannot work aerobically straightaway as it takes time to switch the aerobic system on. If we start intense exercise without a warm-up, the aerobic system does not have enough time to switch on; we therefore have to provide energy anaerobically, with resultant lactic acid formation.

The function of a warm-up is to 'switch on' the aerobic system and allow the body to reach a steady state where the energy provided by the body exactly matches its requirements through exercise. Once this is done, less waste is produced and so our recovery after exercise will be much faster.

Mechanical effects

The mechanical effects of warm-up occur as a direct result of tissue heating. Chemical reactions involved in the production of energy for the working muscle and the removal of waste products are speeded up with warmth. In addition, nerve impulses travel faster when a nerve is warm. The effects of a warm-up on nerve conduction is particularly important for the speed of reflexes, which protect the muscles from injury.

When a substance is heated it becomes more pliable, and this is exactly the same for the body tissues. We have seen that there is a relationship between load and deformation of a tissue (*see* fig 1.11). One of the effects of warm-up is to move the load–deformation curve to the right. This means that, for any given load, a warm tissue will be elastic for longer and will reach its failure point later. The effect of these changes is to make stretching exercises both more effective and safer. In addition, the fluid within a joint becomes less stiff (viscous) when warm so the joint will move more smoothly.

Figure 4.1 shows the effect of heat on a tendon as it is stretched. Because tissues will stretch more easily after a warm-up, it is important that stretching exercises are not performed at the beginning of a warm-up period. Vigorously touching the toes will not act as a warm-up for the hamstrings, and may tear them instead!

> **Key point**: Warm up enables the body to reach a 'steady state' of energy production gradually, and makes tissues more pliable and ready to exercise.

Psychological effects

Two effects are important here: *arousal level* and *mental rehearsal.*

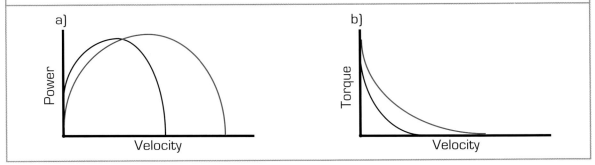

Figure 4.1 Vertical jump test – effect of tissue temperature increase due to a warm-up: (a) peak power increases, demonstrated by the increased height; (b) maximum velocity of shortening increases, and torque–velocity curve shifts to the right from Enoka, 1994

Arousal level

There is a direct relationship between arousal and performance, and this can be illustrated on the *human performance curve* (*see* fig 4.2). Initially, as arousal increases, so does performance. However, after a certain point an individual becomes too aroused (they are now 'stressed') and their performance suffers. As an illustration of this mechanism, imagine you have had a boring day and you arrive at the gym not really wanting to exercise. Your arousal level is low so your exercise performance will be poor. If you then go into an exercise class, however, the instructor, the music and the other people will increase your arousal level. You feel motivated and your exercise performance improves. On the other hand, imagine you are an athlete competing in an important game and you miss a shot that normally you would find very easy. Perhaps you are nervous, your heart is pounding and your arousal level is too high, so your performance suffers.

The function of a warm-up should be to place an individual at the optimum point on the human performance curve; this will change depending on the individual and the sport. A person who is very introverted and under-aroused may need to

be 'psyched up' in a warm-up to move them to the right on the curve. Someone who is aggressive, extrovert and 'hyperactive' may need to be calmed down and moved further to the left on the curve. Events that require highly skilled movements tend to be performed better at lower levels of arousal when an individual is calm and can focus his or her attention. Events that require power or explosive actions are normally performed better when higher levels of arousal are achieved. This is why stretching exercises are

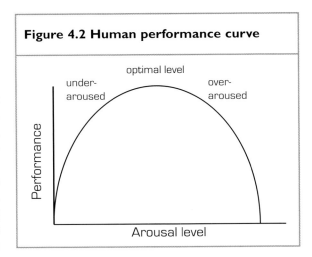

Figure 4.2 Human performance curve

best performed after a gentle but thorough warm-up to heat the body tissues, but relax the mind.

> **Key point:** A good warm-up will make a person optimally aroused for sport. An anxious individual should be calmed down and an under motivated individual should be 'psyched up'.

Mental rehearsal

The second psychological effect of a warm-up is that of mental rehearsal. Complex actions tend to be forgotten between exercise bouts. The first or second repetition of a complex action may not be as good as the fourth or fifth, when you have had time to 'get into' the movement. With skilled actions, it is essential that we rehearse the movement, slowly going through a golf swing, for example, before we perform the action at full speed. This is very important with activities that require a high degree of active flexibility, such as dance and martial arts.

Types of warm-up

A warm-up can either be '*passive*', with the body heated from the outside, or '*active*', using exercise to form the heat internally. An example of a passive warm-up is to have a sauna or hot shower. An active warm-up can be achieved through gentle jogging or using light aerobics. Both types can be effective, but are appropriate in different situations.

An active warm-up is the type normally used before exercise, while the passive warm-up is useful when stretching a muscle tightened from a previous strain. The advantage of the passive warm-up, from the point of view of injury, is that it does not require the athlete to move the injured tissues in order to create body-heat. The use of external heat can also reduce pain and

muscle spasm, helping the muscle to relax and allowing the stretch to be taken further.

In addition to active and passive types, a warm-up may also be either *general* or *specific*. A general warm-up, such as jogging or static cycling, will affect the whole body. The effects here are mainly on the major body systems such as the heart, lungs and blood vessels. This should be followed by a specific warm-up concentrating on the body-part and action to be used in a particular exercise. The effects now are more localised, mainly affecting body tissues used in the actual exercise and rehearsing the action to be performed (*see* fig 4.3).

Warm-up techniques

The amount of exercise required for an effective warm-up will depend very much on a person's fitness level and the exercise to be performed in the main part of the workout. This is because changes in body temperature vary with body-size, fat level and rate of body metabolism. In addition, sports differ tremendously in the demands they make on the body tissues, so a warm-up before a vigorous game of hockey would clearly need to be more extensive than one for a casual game of bowls. Equally, a top-level sprinter will require a more thorough warm-up session than a casual sportsman or woman, because the sprinter is likely to be able to push him or herself to a higher physical level. The following are guidelines.

- **Intensity:** If it is to be effective, a warm-up must be intense enough to cause mild sweating. When this happens, it indicates that the inside (core) temperature of the body has increased by about 1°C. Increasing the core temperature by this amount has been shown to be the minimum requirement for bringing about the warm-up changes discussed above.

Figure 4.3 Types of warm-up

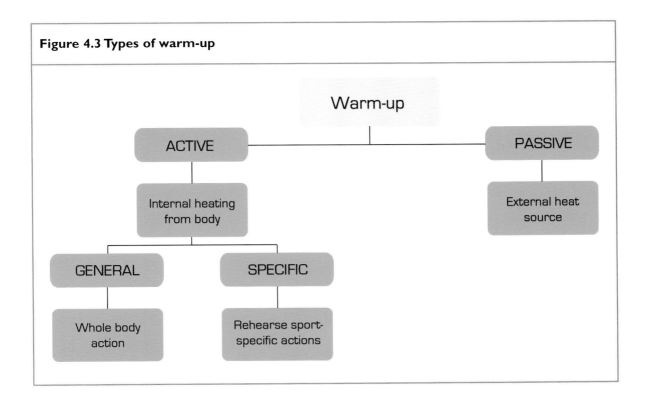

- **Clothing:** Because we are trying to raise the body temperature, it is best to perform the warm-up wearing warm clothing to keep the body-heat in. The amount of clothing needed to provide adequate insulation will depend largely on the outside temperature. Light clothing may be suitable in a warm sports-hall, but thick fleecy material with a weatherproof covering layer will be needed on the touch-line of a cold and windy pitch.
- **Activities:** Warm-up activities should be continuous and rhythmical in nature. Gentle jogging, light aerobics, or cycling on a static bicycle in the gym are all examples of good warm-up activities. Once light sweating has begun, the major joints should be taken through their full range of movement, starting with small movements which gradually become larger. Finally, some sport-specific actions must be included in the warm-up period as a part of skill rehearsal.
- **Time:** A good warm-up may take 10–15 minutes, but it is time well spent. Note that we are using a warm-up before stretching rather than using stretching as part of a warm-up. This makes sense because tissues will stretch more effectively when warm. The movements we use in the warm-up to take the major joints through their range of motion are not stretching exercises as such. The warm-up movements take the joints through their full range of motion, but do not try to increase this range of motion as stretching exercises would.

Key point: Match your warm-up to your body requirements and exercise type and intensity.

Table 4.1	Overload components		
Type	Intensity	Duration	Frequency
Fitness component ('S' factor)	How hard	How long	How often

Warm-down

Just as it is vital to begin an exercise session slowly by warming up, so it is important to end it the same way by using a warm-down or cool-down. The warm-down period has a number of important effects.

First, during intense exercise the heartbeat increases, and the beating of the heart is actually helped by the contraction of the exercising limb muscles. As these muscles contract they squeeze the blood vessels that travel through them, thus helping the blood to return to the heart. If an individual stops exercising suddenly, the limb muscles no longer pump the blood vessels and help the heart. The demand placed on the heart is increased and the pulse will actually get faster even though exercise has stopped.

An effective warm-down can also reduce muscle ache. This is caused partly by lactic acid formation, and partly through tiny muscle tears that occur during very hard training. Hard training causes local swelling within a muscle, giving *delayed onset muscle soreness* (DOMS). In the case of DOMS, you feel fine the day after a workout, but the day after that you feel stiff. To reduce these effects you should perform a warm-down using similar exercises to those chosen for the warm-up, gradually lowering the exercise intensity until resting levels are reached. It is interesting to note that stretching exercises may be used to reduce muscle pain that occurs after intensive strength training.

Finally, shake your muscles to loosen and relax them, and take a warm shower to flush fresh blood through them and aid recovery. Because blood is still needed in the muscles after exercise in order to aid recovery, you should not eat a large meal immediately. If you feel hungry and in need of an 'energy boost' eat a small amount of sweet, high-carbohydrate food such as a banana or a piece of toast and honey.

> **Key point:** When planning your workout, allow at least 5 minutes for a warm-down. Do not fill all your time with hard exercise and then rush out of the gym.

Overload

To achieve a training effect, the body must be exposed to a physical stress that is greater than that encountered in everyday living. If this is done the body is said to be *overloaded*, and the body tissues will change or 'adapt' as a result, provided they are given time to do so. The two key points regarding overload are: that the overload must be greater than that normally encountered by the body; and that time is needed for the body tissues to adapt. Tissue adaptation of this type can be illustrated by something rubbing on the skin, such as a stone in a shoe. If the rubbing occurs continuously (without rest), the skin will break down and bleed. If, however, the rubbing occurs and then the skin is rested before being stressed again, a hard callus will form. In the former case, no recovery period was available for tissue adaptation, in the latter, tissue adaptation (callus growth) occurred in the recovery period itself. Exactly the same occurs with exercise.

If we take weight training as an example of this process, the resistance from the weight causes muscle breakdown. The body overcompensates by building stronger muscle in the rest period between exercise. For this reason, rest is vital, and intense exercise should not be practised every day, but on alternate days.

As fitness improves, exercise must become harder so the body continues to be taxed to the same degree. If the body has adapted to the training load, further improvement will only occur if the training intensity is increased. Exercise must therefore be progressive (gradually getting harder) for the overload to have the same effect.

Overload has four components: type, intensity, duration, and frequency (*see* table 4.1).

- **Type:** The training type will dictate the tissue changes that will occur, and the training is said to be 'specific'. For each of the components of fitness (*see* table 4.2) a different training type is required. When training for stamina the intensity of exercise may be determined by the pulse rate, and when training for strength by the weight lifted.
- **Intensity and duration:** Training must be intense enough to challenge the body tissues, and of sufficient duration for the challenge to continue long enough. The intensity of flexibility training may be assessed by the range of movement and how long the stretch is held.
- **Frequency:** The frequency must be appropriate – often enough for the tissues changes to build up, but not too often so that recovery is allowed.

The American College of Sports Medicine (ACSM) defined the appropriate overload for health-related exercise in 1978, and this was updated in 1990 and again in 2002. They say that the quality and quantity of exercise required to maintain aerobic fitness and body composition is a training frequency of three to five days per week at an intensity of between 60–90 per cent of the age-related maximal heart rate. This should be carried out for 20–60 minutes each time and be rhythmical or continuous in nature. Resistance training should be performed for one set of 8–12 repetitions of 8–10 exercises for the major muscle groups for two days per week, and involve both machine and free weight exercise.

From the point of view of stretching, the ACSM says: '*Flexibility exercises should be incorporated into the overall fitness programme sufficient to develop and maintain range of motion (ROM). These exercises should stretch the major muscle groups and be performed a minimum of 2–3 days a week. Stretching should include appropriate static and/or dynamic techniques. . . . Static stretches should be held for 10 to 30 seconds. . . . PNF techniques should include a 6 s contraction followed by 10 to 30 s assisted stretch.*' So, the general advice for stretching is to stretch on a regular basis and hold the stretches for longer than has traditionally been used in sport (see chapter 6, Stretching research). In addition, the effects of a warm-up make it desirable to perform a warm-up before stretching if the aim is to improve range of motion (developmental stretching). However, if the aim is simply to maintain the range of motion (maintenance stretching), the stretches themselves may form part of the warm up or exercise programme.

> **Key point**: General guidelines for stretching are to: (a) stretch the major joints and two-joint muscles 3–5 times per week; (b) hold each stretch for 20–30 s; and (c) stretch after a warm-up of sufficient intensity to induce light sweating.

Training effects

We have seen that an overload on body tissue gives a training effect. This effect is largely reversible, however. If training stops, the benefits achieved for each fitness component will be lost and 'detraining' will occur.

In just 20 days of total rest, stamina reduces by 25 per cent – a loss of about 1 per cent per day. Strength reduction is even greater, with average losses over the same period of 35 per cent. Muscles that have become more flexible with training will slowly tighten again, and muscle imbalance may occur if some muscles tighten more quickly than others (*see* page 54). Skill-based components including sports technique, balance and co-ordination last longer, but will gradually degrade with time. The principle is clear – 'use it or lose it!'

Training has immediate, short-term and long-term effects.

- Immediate effects are the body's responses to exercise. These are brought about by increased metabolism and include higher heart and breathing rates, changes in blood flow, increased body temperature, and chemical alterations to enzymes within the working muscles.
- Short-term training effects become apparent when exercise stops and the body tries to reduce its metabolic rate to resting levels once more. Body temperature has increased, so sweating continues to try to cool the tissues. Energy has been used and must be replaced, so breathing rate and heart rate remain high. Waste products have been formed as energy was 'burnt', and these wastes must be eliminated.
- Long-term effects are the cumulative results of exercise, reflecting the body's adaptation to training. Intense training stresses the body; over time, the body learns from this and changes so that the next training bout will not stress it as much. If a training session is not intense enough, it will not stress the body sufficiently and no adaptation will occur. However, if it is too intense and the body cannot cope, injury may result. Following training, time must be allowed for the body to change and adapt, so rest for recovery from exercise is vital.

Components of fitness

It is generally accepted that two types of fitness exist: health-related and task- (performance) related. These include various components which can be described as 'S' factors for convenience (*see* table 4.2). Health-related fitness includes components that are considered to be beneficial to health. In this context the term *stamina* is used to encompass both heart–lung fitness and muscle endurance. This fitness component is important to the health of the heart and circulatory system. *Suppleness* (flexibility) and *strength* are concerned with the health of the musculo-skeletal system, and are important in injury prevention.

These three components are all essential to sports performance, but in addition *speed* and *skilled action* are required. Speed involves rapid muscle contraction and the elastic abilities of the muscle and is important for explosive events.

Table 4.2	Fitness components ('S' factor)
Stamina	Cardiopulmonary and local muscle endurance
Suppleness	Active, passive, PNF
Strength	Concentric, eccentric, isometric
Speed	Speed (rate of movement), power (rate of doing work)
Skill	Balance and co-ordination
Specificity	Exercise must match required training outcome
Spirit	Psychological factors of training

Skill includes the skills needed for a particular sport, as well as general skills such as balance and co-ordination.

Injury will be more likely if the fitness components become unbalanced. For example, an inexperienced bodybuilder may have excessive strength in comparison with their flexibility, making muscle pulls more likely. A poorly trained distance runner may have a lot of stamina to protect the heart, but very little strength or flexibility, leaving the joints open to injury. Many keep-fit enthusiasts see themselves as 'very fit' because they may be strong and supple and have plenty of stamina, but endless hours spent working on gym machines will do little to improve skill, and fitness enthusiasts can be left clumsy with poor balance and co-ordination ability. So the message is clear: an overall training programme must work on **all** the fitness components if it is to be totally effective.

Specificity

Over a period of time, the demands placed on the body during exercise cause the body to change. With stretching, the muscles become more flexible; with weight training they become stronger; and with running, stamina improves. These changes are the adaptations to exercise and will closely match the type of demand placed on the body. For example, running marathons will improve aerobic endurance, while sprinting will build anaerobic power. If we wanted to improve our distance-running ability there would be little point in using sprint training, because the body adaptation that would occur would not be the right one.

SAID principle

The above example illustrates an important principle, that of *training specificity*. We can say that all

training follows the SAID principle: 'specific adaptation to imposed demand'. Put simply, this dictates that the change that takes place in the body (the adaptation) will closely resemble (be specific to) the type of training used (the imposed demand).

Applying this principle to stretching means that, when choosing stretching exercises to improve sports performance, we must match the range of motion, the muscles stretched, and the muscle balance around a joint to similar actions in the desired sport. For example, if a soccer player needs stretching exercises, these can be designed for the muscles used in kicking. The exercises should take account of any tightness a player may already have, and the stretching programme should be individually designed. Also, stretching should be applied as part of a general training programme, so that increases in flexibility are matched by strength improvements, which enable the player to control the new range of motion that he or she has gained.

Flexibility training

What stops a joint moving through an infinite range of motion?

We need to look at two areas to explain this: internal (body) factors and external (environmental) factors.

One important internal factor is bone. Obviously, we cannot affect the amount of bone in a joint, but we must be aware of it as a limiting factor to flexibility. After a fracture, for example, the amount of bone will increase over the fracture site. If this area is near a joint, range of motion may be reduced: in this case it would be fruitless to continue a stretching programme to this region. Equally, an elderly athlete may have osteoarthrosis, a condition in which the bone surfaces of the joints become uneven and more bone is formed. Again, the bone itself may limit movement and it would be dangerous to attempt any forceful stretching manoeuvres. Soft tissues such as tendons, ligaments, the joint capsule and the skin itself will limit movement. These tissues are *inert*, i.e. they do not contract. However, they do have elastic properties so they will stretch. Muscle is also an important factor: it is contractile and its contraction is governed by a number of important reflexes. Surrounding the muscle, however, is a connective tissue framework that will limit movement, so a muscle may be seen as both an inert and contractile structure.

The most important external factor that affects flexibility is temperature. When warmed, the body tissues become more pliable. A thorough warm-up must, therefore, be performed before stretching exercises are attempted. Often, vigorous stretching exercises are performed as a warm-up, which is incorrect: until the tissues are warm, and an athlete starts to sweat lightly, full-range stretching exercises should not be attempted. In the same way that warm tissue is more pliable, cold tissue is stiffer. Research has shown that when stretching is used after injury, a greater range of motion can be achieved if the muscle is cooled with ice while holding it in its final stretched position.

Individual differences in flexibility

If you ask the members of any class to perform a stretching exercise, you immediately see a tremendous variation in movement: some will be more flexible than others; some will move into the position in a smooth and effortless way; while others will stumble clumsily into the exercise. The differences reflect variations in both range of movement and skill-level between individuals.

Individuals involved in strength and power events are usually less flexible than those who use their own body-weight as resistance, such as swimmers, gymnasts and dancers. The degree of flexibility depends also on whether a person's fitness programme is balanced. Inexperienced bodybuilders who just train for strength and bulk are among the least flexible, while teenage girl gymnasts can be among the most flexible.

Females are generally more flexible than males, especially around the hip and shoulder. Hormonal changes will also affect flexibility in females. During pregnancy, and to a lesser extent during menstruation, *relaxin* hormone is released into the bloodstream. This, together with progesterone and oestrogen, has the effect of relaxing the pelvic ligaments, and making the joint between the base of the spine and the pelvis (the sacroiliac joint) more mobile. The effects of hormone changes may remain for as long as six months after pregnancy, so during this time the individual is at risk from rapid end-range stretching exercises.

Range of movement is also dictated by lifestyle and previous injury. Inactive individuals who get the exercise message late in life will be inflexible, and in many cases the range of movement they gain will never be as great as the range they could have achieved had they been active all their lives. In addition, the limitation to range of movement can often be permanent, dictated by years of poor posture and faulty movement techniques. Previous injuries can leave a reduced range of movement as the only outward sign that problems have occurred. Individuals with a history of low back pain will often be tight in the lower spine and hamstring muscles, while those with shoulder problems may be left with limited shoulder rotation movements. In cases where an individual's flexibility is asymmetrical (greater on one side of the body than the other), a flexibility programme must aim to restore symmetry and not just increase range of movement.

Flexibility and body type

Each of us has a different type of body: some are fatter, some are thinner, and some are more or less muscled. The degree to which we differ can be partially explained by our 'body type' or *somatotype*. Three extreme body types are recognised: *mesomorphs* (muscular); *endomorphs* (fatter); and *ectomorphs* (thinner) (*see* fig 4.4).

- **Mesomorphs** have more bone and muscle development. Their bodies are made for strenuous physical activity, and individuals of this type tend to be heavily muscled. The chest is broad, and the shoulders are wider than the waist – the 'Tarzan' type.
- **Endomorphs** have rounder physiques and they tend to put on and store fat. They have a 'pear drop' appearance with the abdomen being as large or larger than the chest – the typical 'Billy Bunter' character.
- **Ectomorphs** have long delicate limbs – the traditional 'bean-poles'.

In reality, few people have physiques that fall firmly into just one of these categories. We are all a mixture of the three extremes. By taking height, weight, bone size, limb girth and body-fat measurements, an individual can be given a score indicating the proportion of each body-type component present in their physiques.

Scores range from 1 to 7, and are presented in the order endomorph/mesomorph/ectomorph. Thus a highly endomorphic individual would score 7/1/1 and a high mesomorph 1/7/1. The somatotype rating can be illustrated graphically so that somatotype averages for different sports can be compared (*see* fig 4.5). We can see, for example, that both gymnasts and basketball players have a high degree of mesomorphy, but that the basketball players have a greater tendency to endomorphy than do the gymnasts. Bodybuilders are highly mesomorphic, as we would expect. Both ballet dancers and swimmers are roughly average on all scores, possibly reflecting the fact that these athletes use their own body-weight as resistance.

Physiological effects of stretching exercise

Most people would recognise that stretching exercises make you more flexible. In other words, you are able to stretch further because your range of motion is greater. In addition, it is a common observation that with stretching, movements

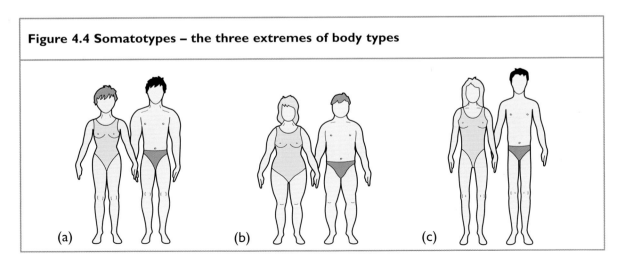

Figure 4.4 Somatotypes – the three extremes of body types

(a)   (b)   (c)

Figure 4.5 Elite athlete somatotypes

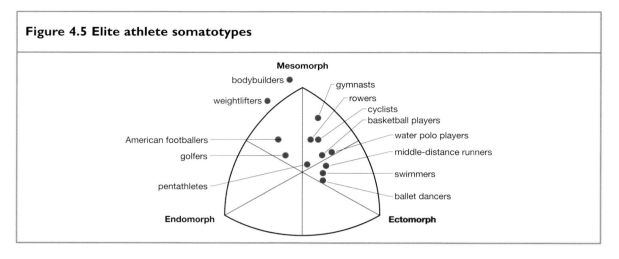

seem somehow easier to perform. What are the mechanisms that achieve these changes?

Habituation

One of the first changes to occur in stretching is an alteration in the stretch reflex. When a muscle is stretched rapidly, its tone increases as a result of the stretch reflex. This is a protective mechanism designed partly to prevent the muscle from getting injured if it is pulled suddenly, but, more importantly, it is part of a postural mechanism called a saving reaction. Because we stand on two feet rather than four, our base of support is very small compared to our height. If you consider a closed-up step ladder, it balances on two feet and is about 5 or 6 feet tall. This is similar to a human. Place the step ladder on its end, however, and it will fall over; not so with the human. The reason that we do not fall is, for the main part, due to the stretch reflex. As we begin to topple forwards, our feet are pushed into dorsiflexion at the ankle and our calf muscles stretched. A stretch reflex occurs in these muscles and they contract to press the toes into the floor and prevent us from falling. As the toes press into the floor, we begin to fall backwards, but once again a stretch reflex occurs to prevent this. At any one time, dozens of stretch

reflexes are taking place to stop us from falling and we sway backwards, forwards and side-to-side in a constant battle with gravity. This continuous movement is called *postural sway*.

So, the stretch reflex is a protective mechanism that increases muscle tone. When we are performing stretching exercises, however, we can override this to actually reduce muscle tone. If we stretch the muscle over and over again, eventually the reflex becomes dulled or 'desensitised' and will not respond to the stretch to the same extent. The process of desensitising the stretch reflex in this way is called *habituation*. It requires repeated stimulation with the same stimulus to improve; in other words, the stretch must be rhythmical (pulsing) rather than haphazard.

> **Key point**: Habituation is the reduction and eventual loss of a response or sensation as a result of continuous stimulation with a constant stimulus.

The point at which the stretch reflex occurs is known as the 'threshold' (*see* fig 4.6). The threshold is higher after repeated stretching, meaning that the muscle can be stretched to a greater range before the stretch reflex occurs.

Figure 4.6 Habituation of the stretch reflex during stretch exercise

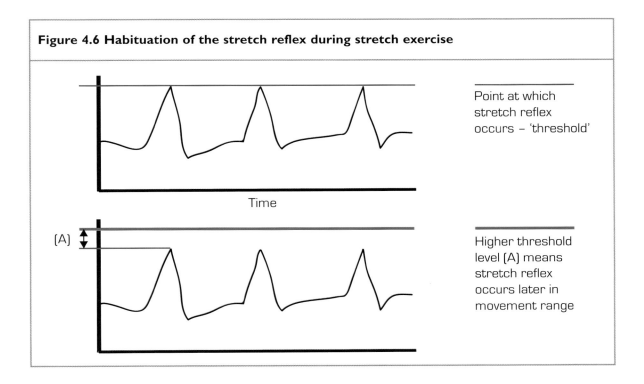

Time

Point at which stretch reflex occurs – 'threshold'

[A]

Higher threshold level [A] means stretch reflex occurs later in movement range

Stiffness changes

When a muscle is stretched, it will pull back using *elastic recoil.* This is the same as for any substance: for example, if we stretch an elastic band it will recoil. Similarly, if we try to stretch a piece of string it will also recoil, but to a lesser extent than the elastic band. This is because the string is less elastic than the band, and therefore more rigid, or stiffer. Because it is stiffer, the string offers more resistance to the stretching movement than the elastic band. To make the string stretch further, we would have to reduce its stiffness and, in so doing, its resistance to motion. This process is exactly what happens with muscle. When a muscle is stretched, it resists the stretch because it has a certain stiffness, which is somewhere between the elastic band and the string. With repeated stretching, however, its stiffness reduces. The process that is occurring here is a little like warming putty.

Stretch putty and it is quite stiff; hold it in your hands and it becomes warm and less stiff, enabling you to stretch it more easily. The same is true of muscle. If you perform a warm-up, the warming of the tissues makes the muscles less stiff and so easier to stretch. Simply by performing a stretching exercise, the same will happen due to the changes in muscle tone that occur. In fact, the stiffness reduction that occurs after a 10 minute period of jogging as a warm-up is exactly the same as that which occurs after 5 repetitions of a static stretch, holding each repetition for 30 s. The reduction in stiffness is about 4–5 per cent following this type of stretching; this may not seem much, but if you imagine the number of steps an athlete takes when running a marathon, for example, you can see that a 5 per cent reduction in stiffness will use less energy and may even reduce the likelihood of injury.

> **Key point:** With stretching, a muscle becomes less stiff and offers less resistance to movement.

Stretch tolerance

Some initial changes in flexibility are seen without an alteration in the electrical signal which comes from the muscle (EMG) due to reflex changes and without a change in muscle stiffness. It seems that the immediate effect of the stretch is an alteration in the amount of discomfort the user is willing to tolerate, or their *stretch tolerance.* The sensation of putting a stretch on a muscle is very intense and, to someone not used to training, this can be interpreted as potentially damaging to the muscle. Feedback systems tend to protect the body from harm, and so any stimulus that is interpreted as a threat will result in a sub-conscious unwillingness to allow the movement to occur. As the pain of the stretch becomes more familiar, rather than being interpreted negatively as a threat, the pain is interpreted positively as a function of training. The individual is therefore more willing to tolerate a greater level of stretch and the resulting greater discomfort; in other words, the individual experiences less pain for the same amount of stretch.

> **Key point:** Stretching causes muscle pain, but over time there is a pain-relieving effect and more stretching can be tolerated.

Changes in muscle sarcomeres

Both changes in muscle tone and muscle stiffness are called *acute* changes, as they occur after relatively short periods of training (months). However, after many years of training, long-term or *chronic* changes may occur. We saw in chapter 3 that muscles contract by using sliding filaments, and that a unit or block of these sliding filaments taken together is called a sarcomere.

As a muscle is contracted, the filaments of the muscle slide together and the sarcomere gets shorter. As the muscle relaxes and is stretched, the filaments move apart and the sarcomere gets longer. This occurs in each sarcomere in the chain right through the length of the muscle. Over a period of time, repeatedly stretching the sarcomeres causes the muscle to adapt by increasing the number of sarcomeres in each of the chains. Because the sarcomeres are lined up one after another (in a series), we call this an increase in *serial sarcomere number* (SSN). This is more commonly seen in individuals who have practised a sport where stretching is an integral part of training, such as ballet.

> **Key point:** Over very long periods, muscle can adept by actually growing longer.

Flexibility methods

We have seen that range of motion can be limited by both inert structures and by the contractile portion of the muscle. Muscle reflexes are important when trying to stretch muscles, while an adequate warm-up is needed to make the tissues more pliable before we stretch. Following a warm-up, the body should be kept warm throughout the stretching period by using warm, loose-fitting clothing such as jogging bottoms and a sweatshirt.

Stretches may be *static,* where no movement is involved, *dynamic,* where the limb is moved as it is stretched, or use *PNF,* a muscle reflex-based technique.

Table 4.3	Stretching types	
STATIC	DYNAMIC	PNF
Pulsing	Active	Contract relax
	Ballistic	CRAC

Figure 4.7 Comparison of stretching techniques

Type	Safety	Ease of application	Effectiveness	Time to apply
static	****	*****	***	****
pulsing	**	***	****	****
dynamic	***	****	*****	**
active	*****	***	****	*****
ballistic	*	***	**	**
PNF				
CR	****	**	****	**
CRAC	****	*	*****	*

These basic types have a number of sub-divisions (*see* table 4.3). Pulsing is an extension of static stretching, active and ballistic are both dynamic movements performed at different speeds, and contract–relax (CR) or CRAC are PNF techniques. The flexibility types are compared in terms of safety, ease of application, effectiveness and time to apply in fig 4.7.

> **Key point:** The three major categories of stretches are static, dynamic and PNF.

Static stretching

Static stretching involves taking a limb to the point at which tightness is felt and holding this position. This is the sort of flexibility used in yoga, for example. As the position is held, the inert structures gradually elongate, while the muscle reflexes detect tension in the muscle tendon and gradually allow the muscle to relax. This is a particularly safe method of stretching, but because the position is held for up to 30 seconds the starting position chosen for the exercise must be comfortable and well supported. Lying and sitting on a mat are good starting positions, but kneeling and single leg standing are not. Once the position is achieved, concentration on breathing out and 'sighing' can allow the muscle to relax further. When the stretch is released, the muscle tension must come off slowly without allowing the tissues to 'spring' back.

Static stretching should generally be applied for 4–5 repetitions, with each stretch being released and the limb rested for 10–20 seconds before the next rep is used. With each rep the range of motion should be seen to gradually improve.

Pulsing

Static stretching is sometimes used with small presses at the end of the range of movement (really moving it into the dynamic category). This is termed *pulsing*, and involves little more than tensing the tissue then releasing it, and repeating this action rhythmically. The repetition causes the muscle reflexes to become accustomed to the stretch and they desensitise (or habituate) to the movement. This process occurs when the body simply gets used to a repeated stimulus and no longer reacts to it. Although this occurs in both ballistic stretching and pulsing, the smaller movements used in pulsing greatly reduce the momentum built up and so the potential for injury is much lower. The down-side of pulsing is that it may not match the high-speed, through-range acceleration used in a particular sport, and so does not provide training specifically for a ballistic sport such as martial arts, for example. It can, however, be built into a programme to greatly reduce the amount of time spent purely on ballistic movement.

Dynamic stretching

Many stretching exercises are used in isolation from other actions and at slow speed. This enables the user to accurately target a particular muscle and is also the best way of avoiding injury, especially for inexperienced exercisers or those returning to stretching after a torn muscle, for example. However, this isolation takes the single muscle action out of the full motor programme of a particular movement. Each movement in sport consists of a number of actions joined together in a chain of movement called a *motor programme*. For example, a jump creates movement (and therefore stretch) at the ankle, knee, hip, trunk and arm. If we simply stretch the calf and achilles, we will increase the flexibility of this region, but only in isolation from the other body-parts and at a speed that fails to match that of the jump action in sport. We could therefore say that slow controlled stretching – although potentially safe and easy to learn – is not truly functional. In other words, using this type of training in isolation will enhance the specific muscle stretch but not the movement performance. This is where *dynamic stretching* comes in.

Dynamic stretching is, literally, stretching with movement. A dynamic stretch is a controlled movement through the full range of motion at either single or multiple joints. Essentially, it involves placing the stretch within the context of a functional action, whether for a specific sport or for daily activities such as lifting. The advantage is that it involves stretching, muscle contraction, muscle control and movement rehearsal (skill and timing). For example, a

dynamic stretch for jumping would be practised at a speed between that of a static stretch (no movement) and that of a full jump (rapid movement). The speed of the movement and the complexity of its action are introduced progressively (*see* fig 4.8) until the action is eventually practised at full functional speed. At this point, a dynamic stretch has often progressed to full plyometric training (*see* page 33). A comparison of some of the features of static and dynamic stretching is shown in table 4.4.

Active stretching

Active stretching is a slower-speed version of classic dynamic stretching. It involves an active contraction (isometric or concentric) of one muscle to its full inner range, requiring the antagonist to stretch fully to its outer range. Active stretching tends to be used as part of a muscle imbalance correction programme and so is *clinically* based, while dynamic stretching is generally used for fitness and sport and so is *performance* based.

Ballistic stretching

Ballistic stretching is similar to dynamic stretching, but is performed at very high speeds and generally to repetition. Two factors are important here. First, when the whole body or trunk is used, the weight of the body moving at speed will build up *momentum*. The energy contained within the momentum can make it impossible to stop the movement soon enough, so tissues can be overstretched and repeated small tears called microtrauma can occur. Over the years this can cause a build-up of scar tissue, altering the mechanics of a joint. Second, the stretch reflex dictates that a rapid stretch will cause muscles to contract and tighten. Instead of increasing range of motion, the range may then actually reduce. It becomes obvious that this type of stretching can be both dangerous and ineffective in many situations.

Figure 4.8 Example of progression of a dynamic stretching for jumping

Static stretch of calf/Achilles and rectus femoris

⬇

Static stretch of calf/Achilles combined with rectus femoris

⬇

Dynamic slow-speed stretch from half-squat position to full standing

⬇

Dynamic mid-/half-speed stretch, as above

⬇

Dynamic slow-speed stretch from full-squat position to full standing

⬇

Dynamic slow-speed stretch, as above, with small jump

⬇

Dynamic fast-speed stretch with larger jump

⬇

Full plyometric action to repetition

However, ballistic stretching can have an important role when carried out under the supervision of a physiotherapist after injury. The reason is that many sports, such as the martial arts, actually involve full-range actions and a high degree of flexibility. If the actions are performed slowly they are dynamic flexibility actions, but when performed explosively – as they often are competitively – they become ballistic actions. The athlete practising this sport does not get injured each time he kicks, simply because he has trained his body to re-set the stretch reflex so that it does not occur at the speed at which he is kicking.

If the athlete should suffer an injury, however, he must regain lost strength and flexibility and gradually reintroduce ballistic flexibility before attempting competitive sport once more. This must be done in a highly controlled and supervised manner. Initially, only mid-range movements are used, then gradually the range of motion is increased over many training sessions. It must be emphasised that full static, active and PNF flexibility, and full strength and power, should be regained before any ballistic actions are used. The danger comes when inexperienced athletes try to copy a person who has been training with this type of action for many years. The body of the inexperienced athlete has not had time to adapt itself to these highly specialised actions, so injury is the frequent outcome.

PNF stretching

PNF (proprioceptive neuromuscular facilitation) stretching is a method adapted from physiotherapy treatment of patients who have had strokes. It involves a series of movements designed to get the maximum out of a muscle by using primitive muscle reflexes.

Table 4.4	Comparison of static and dynamic stretching
Static	**Dynamic**
• Isolates bodypart	• Uses several bodyparts simultaneously
• Able to focus on single structure	• Faster action
• Slow and controlled	• Involves several fitness components
• Uses single fitness component	• Can be used to match functional movement
• Starting position usually fully supported	• Movement rehearsal
• Little skill required	• Skill and timing used

Contract-relax

The first PNF technique is called *contract–relax* (CR). With this method, the athlete must first contract the muscle to be stretched and hold the contraction for 10–20 seconds. During this period the golgi tendon organs will register the tension build-up and cause autogenic inhibition, allowing an increased range of motion to be achieved. Because the muscle is tensed isometrically, this technique is also called *post-isometric relaxation* (PIR) and is also used as part of *muscle energy technique* (MET).

Contract–relax–agonist–contract

The second PNF technique is called *contract–relax–agonist–contract* (CRAC). This consists of the contract–relax method first, but goes further by using the fact that when one muscle contracts, its opposing neighbour (the antagonist) must relax. This reflex, called *reciprocal innervation* (*see* page 32), allows us to stretch still further. To perform the CRAC method, the muscle to be stretched is first contracted and held for 20 seconds. This muscle is then relaxed, a brief pause is allowed, and then the opposing muscle is contracted to pull further into the stretched position. This has the added benefit of strengthening the muscle group that controls the range of motion, but can be difficult for some individuals to practise unsupervised.

General stretching guidelines are summarised in table 4.6.

Starting positions

The starting position for any stretching exercise is important both in terms of safety and effectiveness. It must allow free movement of the part of the body that is to be stretched, and it must be stable. An unstable position can cause an individual to lose balance and, therefore, lose control of a movement, placing excessive strain on the tissues being stretched. In addition, positions that are uncomfortable do not allow individuals to relax completely, and excessive tension in a muscle is not conducive to effective stretching. Furthermore, some individuals with medical conditions will find that certain starting positions, which place excessive or unbalanced stress on a weakened part of the body, are unsuitable. Table 4.5 shows a variety of common starting positions with points to note and suggested modifications.

Use of apparatus

Any form of training requires the body to be overloaded sufficiently to cause an adaptation. In the case of stretching exercises, the overload is to increase the range of motion and hold the position. This is normally achieved manually,

Table 4.5	Starting Positions	
Starting position	**Points to note**	**Modifications**
Standing	Individuals must stand in an erect and balanced posture. Common errors are to stand in a slumped or round-shouldered posture which does not allow correct spinal movement. With the feet together the position is unstable, especially if an individual has poor balance. The body-weight must be taken equally through both legs.	Standing with feet apart (stride standing), or with one foot in front of the other (walk standing), facing the direction of movement. Improve stability further by holding on to an object (support standing).
Walk standing (one foot in front of the other) Step standing (one foot up on a step)	Both positions are more stable than standing alone, but excessive stress may be placed on the knee if leg alignment is not correct. Ensure that the knee passes directly over the middle of the foot on the leading leg.	Use the thigh of the leading leg to lean on for support.
Supine lying	If the hip flexors are tight the pelvis may be tilted forwards, increasing the lumbar lordosis and placing pressure on the lumbar spine (see page 75). In individuals who have little body fat and prominent pubic bones, pressure from a hard floor on body prominences can be painful. Some elderly subjects find lying makes breathing difficult for them, and some with arthritis of the neck joints find lying without a pillow causes dizziness and nausea.	Always lie on a padded mat. Use a rolled towel beneath the lower spine for support. Raise the neck on a small pillow or folded towel for elderly subjects. Bend the knees (crook lying) to relax the hip flexors and reduce pressure on the lumbar spine.
Prone lying	Individuals must turn the head to one side to be able to breathe freely, and this can place excessive stress on the neck if the position	Always use a well-padded mat, and encourage male subjects to press testicles away from compression from the pubic

Table 4.5	Starting Positions cont.	
Starting position	Points to note	Modifications
	is held. Pressure over prominent pelvic bones can be painful, and male subjects may find testicular compression occurs. Those with patellar pain find compression on a hard surface extremely painful.	bone. Place a rolled towel below the forehead to enable the subject to breathe freely without compressing the nose. Bend the knees and place a rolled towel beneath the ankles.
Sitting	When the hips are flexed further than 45 degrees, tightness in the hip tissues begins to tilt the pelvis and flatten the spine. Eventually the spine may round, giving back-pain after prolonged periods. Holding the head too far forwards places stress on the neck and shoulder muscles.	Encourage individuals to 'sit tall' and avoid slumping. Sit with knees apart to allow the pelvis to tilt freely and maintain the lumbar lordosis.
Kneeling	Pressure on the front of the knee is very painful. Kneeling on all fours (prone kneeling) may place stress on the wrist. Kneeling on the knees only (high kneeling) places increased stress on the patella and can be unstable.	Use a well-padded mat. Ensure that the knees are shoulder-width apart to aid stability. Hold on to an object when using high kneeling.

but apparatus may be used. Most commonly, a towel or belt is used to support the part of the body being stretched and to allow greater relaxation. For example, when a subject is quite inflexible, thigh stretches are sometimes easier if a towel is placed around the foot. Belts and pads may be used to keep the spine straight when hip exercises are used, as there is a tendency to allow the spine to round, increasing lumbar stress.

Various machines are available to facilitate adductor stretches in the hope of achieving the classic 'splits' position. These are normally hydraulic or ratchet devices that force the legs further into abduction. From the point of view of safety, the amount of force used and its point of application are of paramount importance. Forcing the hips into an abducted position can place an excessive stress on the hip tissues. Applying this force below the knee can stress the medial ligament of the knee by imposing an inward (valgus) stress on these structures.

Continuous passive motion (CPM) machines have been used in a hospital setting for a number of years, and these are now being seen in the sporting context. The machines are electrically powered, and move the joints through a specified range for a set period. The amount of force

Table 4.6	Stretching guidelines
Stretching type	Technique
Static	• Take limb to end of range • Hold for 20-30 seconds
Pulsing	• Take limb to end of range and stop • Perform 10-20 small amplitude (2-3 cm) presses
Dynamic	• Take limb through full range of motion combining several movement planes (e.g. flexion/abduction/rotation) • Mimic sports actions
Active	• Take limb to end of range by contracting opposite muscle maximally • Use to correct muscle imbalance
Ballistic	• Perform repeated vigorous full-range action used in sport • Practise at competition speed
CR	• Contract muscle to be stretched against partner-applied resistance • Relax, and then apply static stretch using partner to guide limb
CRAC	• Contract muscle to be stretched against partner resistance • Relax, and then pull limb into stretched position using opposite muscle • Final force supplied by user

available makes it essential that these machines are used only under the direct supervision of a physiotherapist.

Stretching frames are also common. These enable the user to take up a more stable body position and reduce the likelihood of 'wobbling' and potentially falling. Some are simply modifications of the traditional wall bar found in school gyms, while others enable the user to sit and perform a variety of stretches from the sitting position as well as from standing.

Developing agility

We have seen that fitness is composed of a number of components. Of these, flexibility – the ability to obtain a range of motion about a joint – is only one. Agility, by comparison, is the ability to use and control this range of motion. For this reason, good agility requires a number of fitness components: flexibility, strength, muscle endurance, skill, and speed. Agility is thus fundamental to good sports performance.

Agility exercises involve controlled movements through a full range of motion, and may be used individually or in a circuit training format. Examples include movements from dance, ballet, aerobics and gymnastics, together with sport-specific actions requiring a high degree of agility.

Summary

• Warming up has been shown to lessen the number of irregular heart beats and reduce the blood pressure during exercise. It will

also make tissue more pliable and affect psychological arousal.
- During a warm-up the movements to be practised during a workout should be rehearsed.
- Both active (exercise) and passive (heating) warm-ups may be used.
- When the body is exposed to a physical stress greater than the stress experienced in normal everyday activities, it is said to be overloaded.
- In 20 days total rest stamina reduces by 25 per cent and strength by 35 per cent.

- Training specificity means that the change that takes place in the body as a result of exercise will closely match the type of exercise used.
- Stretching achieves its effects by changing muscle reflexes, making muscle less stiff and relieving the pain of the stretch.
- Long term effects of stretching can make a muscle grow longer.
- Three body types exist: mesomorph (muscular), endomorph (fatter) and ectomorph (thinner). We are all a mixture of these three types.
- Stretching may be static, dynamic or PNF.

POSTURE

5

Why is posture important?

Posture is simply the relationship (alignment) between different parts of the body. Posture is important from two standpoints. First, good posture underlies all exercise techniques. Exercises started from a basis of poor posture tend to be awkward and clumsy, with unequal tension placed on some body tissues. This can eventually lead to the accumulation of stress and consequent overuse injuries. Second, postural stress in daily life overworks some tissues and under works others, leading to an imbalance of flexibility and strength. In the short term this imbalance gives rise to postural pain; but in the long term, because joints are pulled out of alignment, altered joint mechanics can lead to the development of joint surface degeneration (*see* fig 5.1).

Posture is maintained by both muscles and non-contractile tissues. A good posture is one in which the different parts of the body are correctly aligned, thus placing the minimum amount of stress on the body tissues. A good posture requires little muscle activity, so it is more relaxed and needs less energy to maintain it. At the same time, joint structures are not overstretched or shortened so much that they cause strain. In both of these cases, a good posture is one that is balanced. It therefore follows that a poor posture requires greater muscle work to maintain it and will almost certainly result in muscle fatigue. In addition, the increased joint-loading forces that result from poor posture increase the likelihood of pain and possible injury.

> **Key point:** Poor posture results in greater muscle work and fatigue as well as well as increased joint loading.

Figure 5.1 Muscle imbalance altering joint mechanics: (a) symmetrical muscle tone – normal joint; (b) unequal muscle pull (imbalance) – joint alignment poor; (c) joint surface degeneration

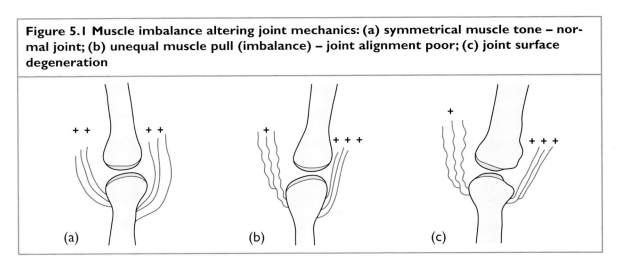

(a)   (b)   (c)

Two types of posture are important. Static posture is that seen at rest, while dynamic posture is that of motion – the type of body position a person takes up when moving. Static posture may be assessed by close inspection of the body, but the study of dynamic posture requires in-depth training, and often the use of advanced laboratory facilities.

A number of factors interact to create a person's static posture. Body type and genetic make-up are important, as are strength and flexibility. In addition, the way a person sees themselves (their body image) and the mental state of an individual will affect their posture.

An individual cannot easily alter their genetic make-up, so the posture with which they were genetically endowed is largely permanent unless surgically changed. Children, for example, who have particular spinal deformities often require a number of complex operations to straighten the spine. Similarly, bone or skeletal 'frame size' is constant for an individual, so a stretching programme must take this into account.

The important factor in the development of both flexibility and strength is *symmetry*. An unequal development of either of these two elements can pull the body out of alignment, causing postural faults.

The balance between postural muscles and movement muscles is also important. Postural muscles hold us up against gravity and include those trunk muscles that give us 'core stability'. Movement muscles will create great power and are able to move rapidly, but will tend to tighten. The combination of tightness (too much tone) of some muscles and sagging (too little tone) of other muscles results in muscle imbalance, which changes our postural alignment and gives rise to postural pain.

Assessing standing posture

From behind

When the body is viewed from behind, with the feet three inches apart, a vertical line should divide it into two equal halves. The pelvic rims (anterior superior iliac spines) should be in the same horizontal plane, and the pubis and pelvic rims should be in the same vertical plane. An individual's posture can be assessed by comparison with a score-chart (*see* table 5.1). Anatomical 'landmarks' are compared with horizontal levels on the right and left sides of the body and include: the knee creases, buttock creases, pelvic rim, angle of the shoulder blades, upper arm bones, ears and skull protuberances. In addition, the alignment of the spinous processes and rib angles is observed. The distance between the arms and the trunk (keyhole), skin creases and unequal muscle bulk are indicators of asymmetrical posture. Slight side bending of the spine (scoliosis) becomes more noticeable when an individual bends forwards (Adam's position) and a marked hump is seen over the twisted ribs.

Looking closely at the shoulder blade (scapula), the inner edge of the blade should be vertical and no more than three finger breadths from the spine. The blade should appear flat against the rib-cage, and no part of it should jut out or appear prominent. The appearance of the shoulder area on the right and left sides of the body should be roughly the same (symmetrical). The bulk of the muscles around the shoulder should be even, with no one area appearing either 'muscle-bound' (excessive bulging) or 'wasted' (hollow). Finally, the contour of the muscle between the shoulder and neck (the upper fibres of the trapezius) should be smooth and rounded, rather than straight and tight like a cord.

Table 5.1	Assessment of standing position from behind
Ear level – hair line	
Shoulder level – cervical spine	
Inferior angle of scapula	
Overall spinal alignment	
Keyhole	
Adam's position	
Skin creases	
Levels of pelvic rim, asis, belt line	
Buttock creases	
Knee creases	
Muscle bulk	
Mid-line	
Achilles angle	
Foot position	

Key point: When looking at a person's posture from behind, symmetry is important. Are both sides more or less equal?

From the side

Standing posture is assessed by comparing it to a plumb-line or vertical line on a wall (*see* fig 5.2). The line begins just in front of the outer

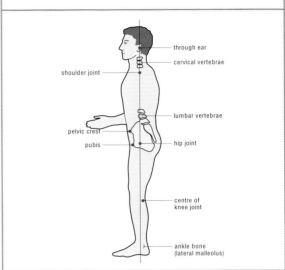

Figure 5.2 Posture plumb-line

through ear
cervical vertebrae
shoulder joint
lumbar vertebrae
pelvic crest
pubis
hip joint
centre of knee joint
ankle bone (lateral malleolus)

ankle bone (lateral malleolus). In an ideal posture, this line should pass just in front of the mid-line of the knee and then through the hip, lumbar vertebrae, shoulder joint, cervical vertebrae and the lobe of the ear. The chest is the furthest point forwards, and the buttocks are the furthest point backwards. The posture is balanced and requires little muscle activity to maintain. When the body moves away from the plumb-line, stress is placed on the body tissues and muscles have to work harder to maintain the unbalanced body position.

Assessing local muscle tightness

The plumb-line posture assessment described above gives us an indication of segmental alignment. From this we can predict which muscles will have poor tone (sag) and which are likely to be tight and require stretching. More precise tests will enable us to be more accurate about which individual muscles are tight, and therefore help us to be more objective with our exercise prescription.

Some of the most frequently used local clinical muscle tests are described below, and further tests are listed in Chapter 15. For all these tests, the client should be positioned ideally on an examination (massage) couch or gym bench. (For more detailed information on postural tests, *see* Norris, 1998.)

Thomas test

The Thomas test measures tightness in the hip flexors (iliopsoas and rectus femoris). The client lies on their back, with their knees bent and hanging over the end of the bench. From this position, both legs are fully flexed, bringing the knees to the chest and flattening the lumbar curve. The client holds one knee to their chest to maintain the lumbar position, and the other leg is lowered towards the horizontal, allowing the knee to extend (*see* fig 5.3). The position of the femur and tibia indicates the muscle tightness.

If the femur rests above the horizontal, the hip flexors are tighter than is desirable. Either the iliopsoas or the rectus femoris could be affected, and straightening the knee will distinguish between the two. If straightening the leg allows the femur to drop down lower, the rectus is the tighter of the two muscles. This is because the rectus works over both the knee and the hip (the iliopsoas does not work over the knee) and straightening the knee takes some of the stretch off the rectus. If the femur position remains unchanged, the iliopsoas is tighter than the rectus.

The knee, hip and shoulder should also be in line. If the femur is abducted, the ilio-tibial band (ITB) is likely to be tight. Similarly the tibia should rest vertically. If it does not, tightness in the hip rotators may be indicated.

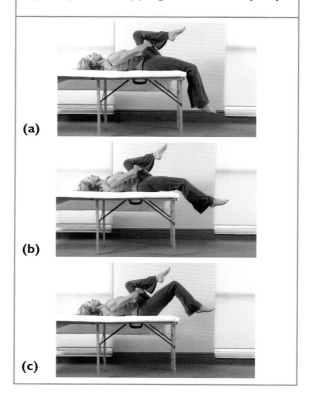

Figure 5.3 Thomas test: (a) knee is gripped to the chest and the opposite leg should touch the couch and show 90° flexion; (b) tight hip flexors; (c) tight abductors (ITB)

(a)

(b)

(c)

Key point: The Thomas test measures tightness in the hip flexors of the lower lying leg. Differentiation can be made between the rectus femoris and the iliopsoas.

Ober test

The Ober test measures tightness in the hip abductors (ilio-tibial band and gluteals) and is named after Frank Ober, who first described it in 1935. Essentially, the test aims to assess the length of the hip abductors while maintaining the

Figure 5.4 Ober test

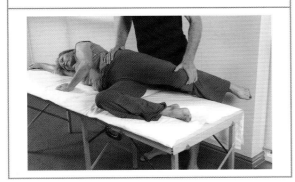

neutral position of the pelvis in the frontal plane. The client lies on a bench on their side with the lower leg bent for comfort. The therapist stands behind them level with their pelvis (*see* fig 5.4). The client's leg is abducted and extended to 15 degrees and the pelvis is stabilised to prevent lateral tilting. The therapist presses down on the client's pelvic rim, with their left hand angling the push towards the client's lower shoulder. The therapist's right hand supports the weight of the abducted upper leg. While preventing any pelvic movement, the upper leg is lowered down, keeping it slightly back. Normally, the leg should lower to the horizontal position before any pelvic movement is detected. In an athlete, the leg should lower to the floor, indicating that the ITB and gluteals possess adequate flexibility. If the leg stops above the horizontal position, or if pelvic movement begins with the leg in this upper position, the ITB is tight. This test is also described in Chapter 11, exercise 102.

> **Key point:** The Ober test measures tightness in the ilio-tibial (ITB) of the upper lying leg.

Tripod test

There are many tests to assess the length of the hamstrings, including the straight leg raise and active knee extension exercises (*see* Chapter 12, exercises 131 and 132). The tripod test, however, measures hamstring tightness and the effect of any tightness on pelvic tilt and low back alignment.

The client sits on the edge of a bench with the feet unsupported. The spine is placed in its neutral position (*see* page 72) with the lower back slightly hollow. From this position, one leg is straightened and the alignment of the lumbo-pelvic area is noted (*see* fig 5.5). Ideally, the leg should be straightened to 70–80 degrees while maintaining spinal alignment. Often, the leg cannot be fully straightened, and the spine sags into flexion, posteriorly tilting the pelvis and flexing the lumbar region. This is important because it indicates that tightness in the hamstrings is dictating spinal alignment which is a common cause of postural back pain. As well as hamstring stretching exercises, core stability exercises should be practised to correct the fault (*see* page 73).

> **Key point:** The tripod test measures the effect of hamstring tightness on sitting posture.

Anterior chest test

Tightness in the pectorals and anterior deltoids will cause the shoulders to be pulled forwards, and is assessed with the client lying on their back. Their arm is taken out to the side into a 'T' position (*see* fig 5.6) and ideally should rest level with the bench. Taking the arm diagonally so that it lies on the horizontal (frontal plane) and at 45 degrees to the spine, will stress the sternal fibres of the pectoralis major and anterior deltoid (*see* fig 5.6(b)). Taking the arm back to the 'T' position and then lowering the arm down the side of the bench will stress the clavicular fibres of the pectoralis major (*see* fig 5.6(c)). In this position, the arm should lie at 70–80 degrees to the chest.

Figure 5.5 Tripod test: (a) pelvis level, leg straightens; (b) tight hamstrings cause backwards pelvic tilt and lumbar flexion

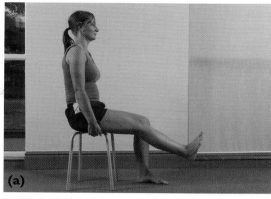

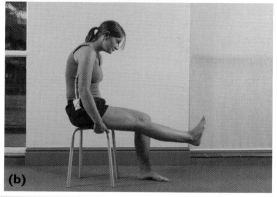

The shoulder can also be pulled forwards by tightness in the pectoralis minor, which attaches from the upper ribs to the corocoid process of the scapula. When this is the case, the back of the shoulder is pulled off the bench in supine lying. Normally, the back of the shoulder should be no more than two to three finger breadths from the bench.

Shoulder adductors

Tightness in the shoulder adductors (lattissimus dorsi and pectoralis major) will limit arm abduction. The latissimus is measured in a supine lying position. The arm is laterally rotated (because the muscle is a medial rotator) and abducted in an attempt to take it behind the ear. Normally, the arm should rest flat on the couch (*see* fig 5.7). Refer to the 'Anterior chest test' for assessment of the pectoralis major.

Postural faults and correction

Enhancing core stability

Before we begin to correct postural faults with stretching, we must ensure that an individual can hold firmly the origin of the muscles to be stretched. If this is not done, when we stretch both ends of the muscle will move and alignment will be poor. Many of the large muscles of the lower limbs attach to the lumbo-pelvic region, while many muscles of the upper limbs attach to the scapula. Both of these areas must be stabilised before stretching begins.

The neutral spine position

The lumbo-pelvic region is stabilised by the deep abdominal muscles (transversus abdominis and internal oblique). Looking at figure 5.8, we can see that the superficial abdominals (rectus abdominis and external oblique) have fibres which run more or less vertically while the deep abdominals have largely horizontal fibres. When the muscles pull, therefore, the superficial abdominals will pull the pelvis to the rib-cage (flexion or rotation), while the deep abdominals will pull the abdominal wall to the spine and 'tighten the girdle'. In this way the deep abdominals are more able to stabilise the trunk and hold it in a 'neutral position' – mid-way between flexion (flat back) and extension (hollow back) (*see* fig 5.9). The neutral position aligns the lumbar tissues optimally and places least stress upon them.

Figure 5.6 Anterior chest test: (a) 'T' position; (b) stressing the sternal fibres of pectoralis major and the anterior deltoid; (c) stressing the clavicular fibres of pectoralis major

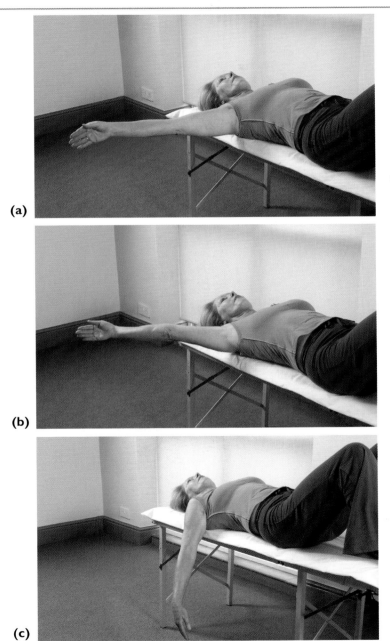

(a)

(b)

(c)

Figure 5.7 Measuring tightness in the latissimus dorsi: full abduction is combined with lateral rotation

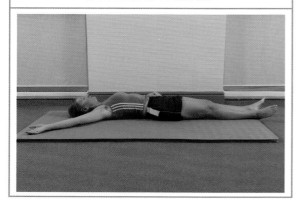

When we move away from the neutral position, stress is increased. As we increase the hollow of the lumbar spine, the facet joints at the back of the spine are compressed. Over time, this can cause pain and joint damage, possibly leading to wear and tear of the joints themselves. If we reduce the hollow in the back, the spine is flexed and stress moves from the facet joints on to the disc. The flexion stress compresses the disc, tending to force it on to the nerves of the lower spine. This type of posture can give pain through nerve compression or nerve entrapment.

Key point: The neutral position of the lumber spine lies mid-way between forward (hollow back) and backward (flat back) tilting of the pelvis.

How to find your neutral spine position

To find the neutral position of the lower spine, we begin standing upright. Tilt the pelvis backwards, forcing your spine to flex (flatten) and then tilt your pelvis forwards, extending (hollowing) your spine. The neutral position is mid-way between fully flattening and fully hollowing the spine. It should be the most comfortable position, depending on your posture type. (Posture types are discussed in detail later in this chapter.)

Figure 5.8 The abdominal muscles

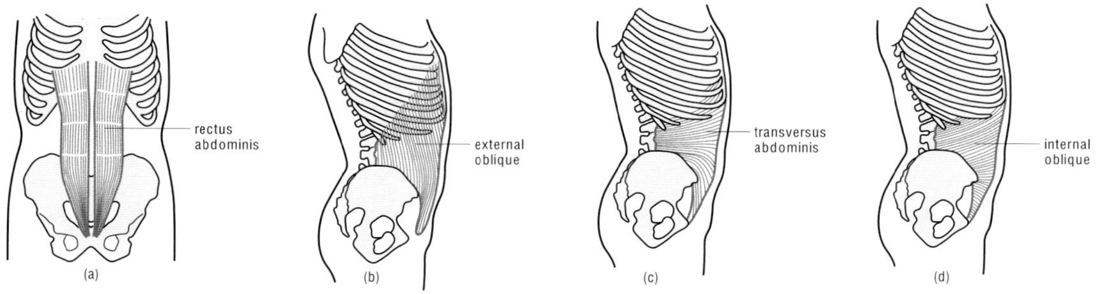

rectus abdominis
(a)

external oblique
(b)

transversus abdominis
(c)

internal oblique
(d)

Figure 5.9 Neutral position of the lumbar spine: (a) neutral positions; (b) hollow back – facet joints compact; (c) flat back – disc is stressed

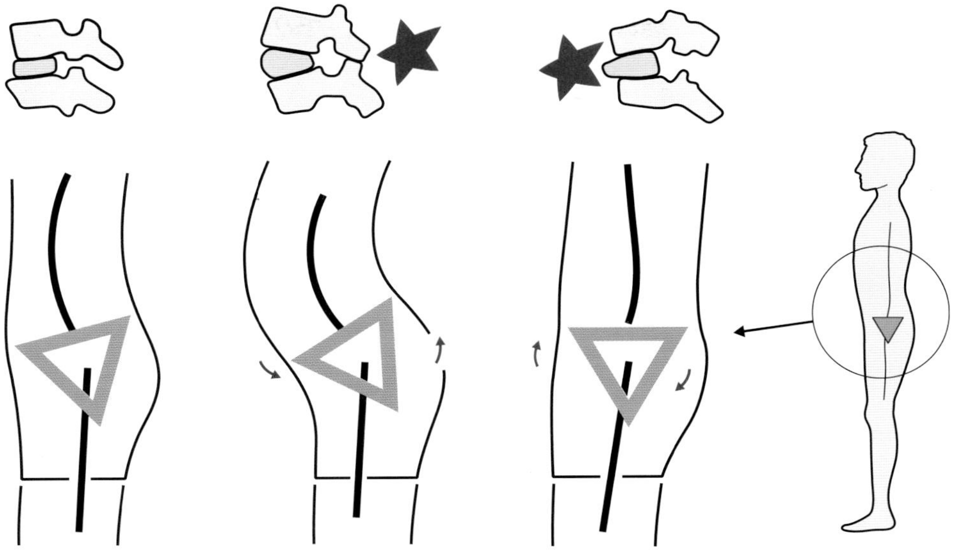

Core stability exercises

Having found the neutral position, we perform a series of simple exercises to re-educate the core stability muscles. First, we have to regain the hollowing function of the abdominals. Many people find this difficult initially, and tend to bend the spine instead.

Abdominal hollowing in standing

Start by standing up straight (*see* fig 5.10). Focus your attention on your tummy button (umbilicus) and tighten your abdominal muscles to pull your tummy button in. A number of faults can occur when performing this exercise (*see* fig 5.11). First, be careful not to take a deep breath or hold your breath, and do not flex the spine. If you look at your lower ribs, they should not move throughout the hollowing action. If the ribs are drawn down, the superficial abdominals are working instead of the deep abdominals. If the ribs lift up, you are simply taking a deep breath and pulling your abdominal wall tight using respiration rather than abdominal muscle action.

Figure 5.10 Abdominal hollowing in standing

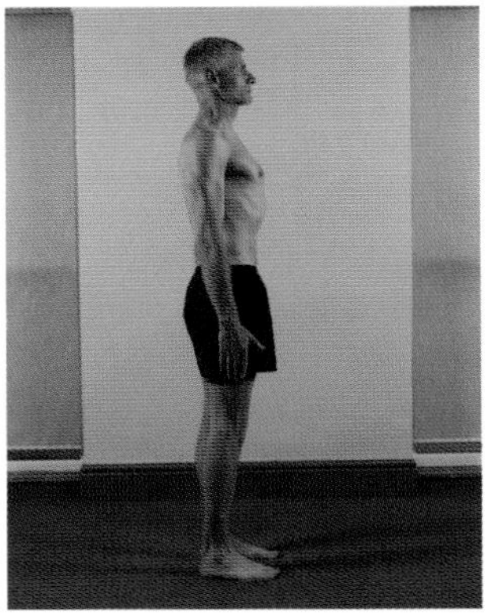

Figure 5.11 Common faults in abdominal hollowing in standing: (a) the distance from the lower ribs to the pelvis (X) remains unchanged; (b) taking a deep breath: the ribs move up, increasing (X); (c) flexing the trunk, the ribs move down decreasing (X)

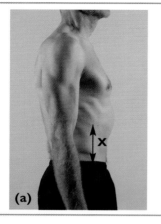

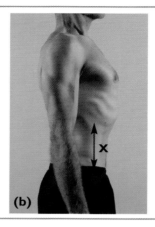

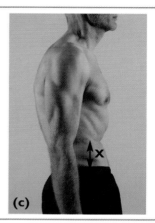

(a) (b) (c)

Abdominal hollowing in kneeling

Allow your abdominal wall to sag down, and then pull it tight and up as if trying to touch your tummy button to your spine. Again, make sure it is only your abdominal wall that is moving. Do not move your spine or hips (*see* fig 5.12).

Heel slide

When you have mastered the abdominal hollowing exercises, you are ready to hold your spine stable against resistance. In the heel slide (*see* fig 5.13), the hip flexor muscles are pulling on your spine, trying to move it away from the neutral position, while you are using your deep abdominal muscles to try to prevent the movement and maintain stability.

Lie down with your knees bent and place your fingertips over your lower abdomen. Pull your lower abdominals tight (hollowing) as before and keep them tight throughout the movement, without holding your breath. Slide one of your legs out straight, making sure that your pelvis does not move and your spine does not hollow. You should aim to perform 10 slow

Figure 5.12 Abdominal hollowing in kneeling

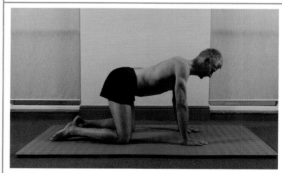

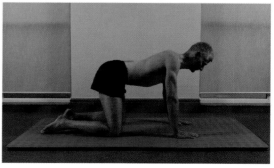

Figure 5.13 Heel slide

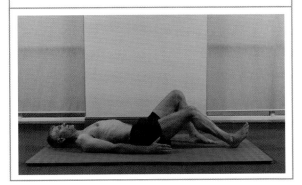

Figure 5.14 The pelvic crossed syndrome (PCS)

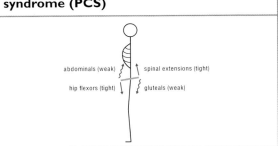

repetitions on each leg, with each complete single leg movement taking about 10 seconds. No pelvic movement at all should occur throughout the whole exercise sequence.

To make it easier to spot unwanted pelvic movement, work with a partner. Place an adhesive marker on the front part of the upper lip of your pelvis (the anterior superior iliac spine) or mark it with a felt-tip pen. This will make it easier for your partner to detect even the smallest amount of pelvic movement.

Hollow-back posture

The lower part of the back (the lumbar spine) should normally be slightly hollow. This curve (the lumbar lordosis) is greatly affected by the tilt of the pelvis. The pelvis is balanced like a see-saw on the hip joints, and is controlled by the abdominal, spinal and hip muscles, and the ligaments that surround these areas. The abdominal muscles, working together with the gluteals and hamstrings, will tilt the pelvis backwards and flatten the lower spine, while the hip flexors and spinal extensors will tilt the pelvis forwards and increase the lumbar curve.

Pelvic crossed syndrome

In many cases an imbalance of these muscles exists, known as the *pelvic crossed syndrome* (PCS). Here we see a combination of excessive length and weakness in the abdominal muscles and gluteals (sagging) and tightness in the spinal extensors and iliopsoas (*see* fig 5.14). The pelvis is seen to tip forwards, pulling the lumbar spine into an increased curvature or lordosis. This, in turn, causes stress to the small facet joints deep within the lumbar spine. This is the classic 'beer belly' posture, also seen after pregnancy and as a result of abdominal surgery.

The weakness of the gluteal muscles has an important bearing on walking and running. Normally, as we take a step and the hip moves into extension, the gluteal muscles contract powerfully to push the body forwards. However, in PCS these muscles are weak and so are unable to propel the body correctly. To compensate for this, the hamstring muscles contract in an attempt to do the work of the gluteals (the hamstrings eventually becoming tight themselves). Because the hamstrings are not as strong as the gluteals, the action of hip extension is weaker. The body tries to make up for this by extending the lumbar spine instead of the hip, and again stress is placed on the lumbar region. The appearance now when running, stepping and walking is of a 'duck waddle' around the pelvic region.

Key point: In the hollow back posture, the abdominal muscles and gluteals are lax (saggy), while the hip flexors and low back are tight.

How to correct the pelvic crossed syndrome

To correct this syndrome, we cannot simply strengthen the gluteal muscles, because the imbalance affects all of the hip muscles. Instead, we must first focus our attention on stretching the tight hip flexor muscles. We saw on page 36 that there is a relationship between antagonistic pairs of muscles: when one muscle contracts, its opposite must relax. In the case of the hip muscles, the tight hip flexors have greater muscle tone and, therefore, may actually reduce the potential tone and strength of the hip extensors that lie opposite. This action of reducing tone by 'inhibition' (fewer nerve impulses reaching the muscle) is also known as *pseudoparesis* and is an important factor in balancing muscle pull around a joint. In the case of PCS, we must stretch the iliopsoas and hamstrings (*see* table 5.2, (a) and (b)) while maintaining a neutral spine position. Once this has been achieved, both the gluteals and the lower abdominal muscles must be re-strengthened to correct the pelvic tilt. It is important to work the abdominals in their inner range to shorten, rather than simply strengthen, the muscles. Details of abdominal work of this type may be found in *Abdominal Training* (Christopher M. Norris, A & C Black, London, 1997).

Kyphotic posture

Upper crossed syndrome

An imbalance pattern also exists around the shoulder girdle, known as the *upper crossed syndrome* (UCS). Here the upper trapezius, levator scapulae and pectoral muscles are tight, while the deep neck flexors and the lower scapular stabilisers (serratus anterior and lower trapezius) are

Table 5.2	Stretching exercises for posture
Problem	Exercise
(a) tight hip flexors	**Iliopsoas:** hold on to an object for stability and press your hips forward
(b) tight hamstrings	**Hamstrings:** hold the back of one leg and straighten it
(c) head appears to be held forward, poking chin	**Chin tuck:** place hand on chin and gently slide head back horizontally
(d) tight band from neck to shoulder (upper trapezius), head appears tilted to one side	**Side bend:** fix the shoulders by gripping a chair and pull the head in the opposite direction
(e) round shoulders	**'pec stretch':** stand in the corner of a room, place the arms on a wall and lean forwards
(f) flat low back	**Low back:** push up on to the elbows
(g) tight back when bending forwards	**Low back:** grip the knees into the chest

Figure 5.15 The upper crossed syndrome (UCS)

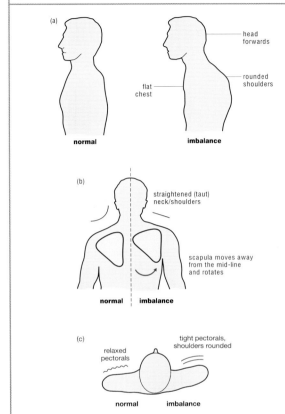

(a) normal / imbalance — head forwards, rounded shoulders, flat chest

(b) normal / imbalance — straightened (taut) neck/shoulders, scapula moves away from the mid-line and rotates

(c) normal / imbalance — relaxed pectorals, tight pectorals, shoulders rounded

spend many hours slumped over a desk and do little exercise in their spare time.

The altered muscular control of the scapulae causes them to twist slightly so that the shoulder socket (glenoid fossa) faces more vertically than normal. This means that the shoulder muscles must work harder to stop the joint from dislocating, and this additional work can give rise to a painful 'frozen shoulder' over time.

Although the shoulder girdle is a separate structure from the thoracic spine, the shoulder posture in UCS pulls the thoracic spine into excessive flexion, forcing the ribs together anteriorly and making breathing more difficult. In some cases, the thoracic vertebrae soften and develop incorrectly, a condition called Scheurmann's disease, which requires specialist treatment. In this case, the shoulder posture results from the spinal posture rather than the other way round.

> **Key point**: In the kyphotic (round shouldered) posture, the chest muscles are tight and short and the shoulder bracing muscles are lax.

How to correct upper crossed syndrome

Just as with the lower limbs, we begin the exercises by improving core stability. This time it is the stability of the shoulder blade (scapula) we are concerned with. It tends to ride up and outwards, and we need to pull it in the opposite direction. The first exercise (*see* fig 5.16(a)) is to sit on a stool and ask your training partner to pull your shoulder into its optimal alignment. The shoulder blade is pulled down and in until its inner edge is vertical and the two blades are about 12–18 cm apart. You 'set' your shoulder muscles to hold this position as your training partner releases the shoulder blade. Try to hold the position for 10–30 seconds. For the next exercise (*see* fig 5.16(b)), you try to correct your own

inhibited and weak. The abnormal posture seen here is one in which the head is held forwards (poking chin) and the normal curve in the neck is flattened out. This head posture places stress on the neck tissues and frequent headaches can result. The shoulders are rounded and the scapulae move further apart. In some cases, the scapulae can be seen standing prominent under the skin (winging). Tightness in the trapezius and levator scapulae is commonly seen as a straightening of the neck/shoulder line, where the muscles stand out like tight cords (*see* fig 5.15). This posture is frequently seen in those who

---

Figure 5.16 Shoulder stability exercises: (a) static reposition; (b) sternal lift

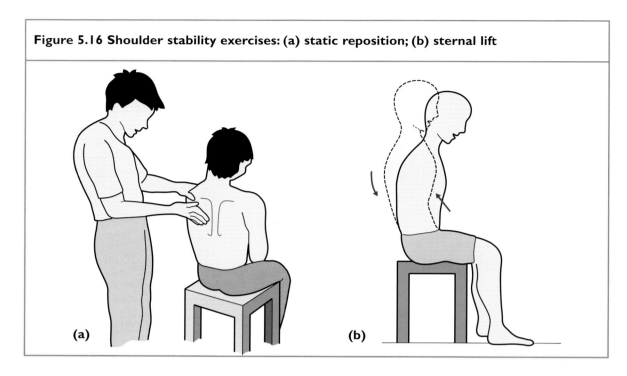

(a)   (b)

---

posture and hold it. Again begin sitting, but try to lift your breastbone (sternum) without taking a deep breath. At the same time draw your shoulder blade in and down. Hold the position for 10–30 seconds as before, breathing normally.

When the kyphotic posture is created by tissue tightness alone, stretching is called for. Stretching is aimed at the neck (*see* table 5.2, (c)), the levator scapulae and upper trapezius (*see* table 5.2, (d)) and the pectoral and anterior deltoid muscles (*see* table 5.2, (e)). In each case, the scapula is stabilised in its optimal position (down and in) throughout the stretch.

In many cases, the lordotic (hollow back) posture and the kyphotic posture may occur together (kypho-lordosis). This is because the increase in the lumbar lordosis results in an increased kyphosis to compensate, which brings the body-weight back over the plumb-line. If this is the case, exercise therapy must be aimed at both areas.

Sway-back posture

In a sway-back posture, the whole pelvis moves forwards and the hips are forced into extension. While the pelvic tilt remains, the thoracic spine flexes and the lumbar lordosis is increased. This stresses the hip ligaments and the ligaments on the front of the lower spine and behind the thoracic spine.

Comparing normal and sway-back postures (*see* fig 5.17), we can see that in the case of normal posture the furthest point forwards is the chest, and the furthest backwards is the buttocks. In the case of sway-back posture, the furthest point forwards is the abdomen and the furthest backwards is the thoracic spine. In the normal posture, the lumbar curve is gently hollow along the whole length of the lumbar spine. In the sway-back posture, the hollow is sharp and more pronounced in the lower area. Finally, in the normal posture the spine and legs are close to the plumb-line, but in the sway-back posture the spine and legs form a curve.

Figure 5.17 Sway-back posture

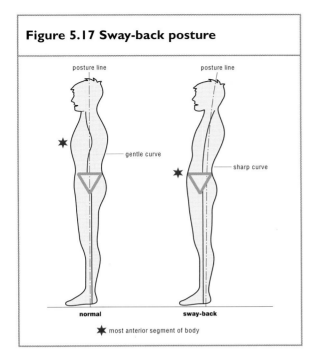

the spine as though you were a puppet on a rope hanging from the ceiling. In addition, the chest should move forwards while the pelvis remains still. The easiest way to learn is by standing in front of a table and imagining the pelvis and chest as two toy building blocks sliding on top of each other (*see* fig 5.18). The hips should not touch the table, and the chest should slide forwards as one unit, without altering spinal alignment.

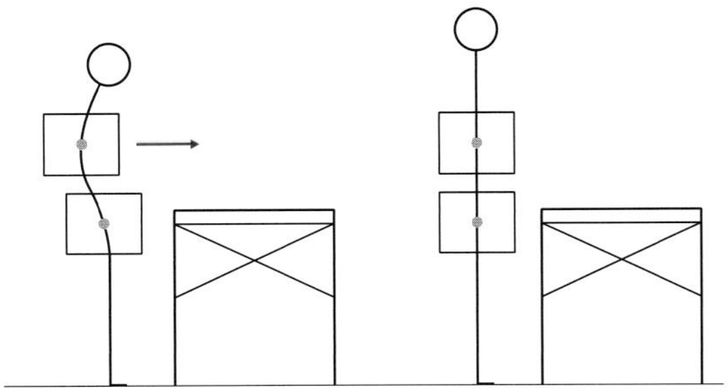

> **Key point:** The sway-back is the 'slouch' posture. The pelvis drifts forwards and the body height is reduced. The key to correction is to 'stand tall'.

The sway-back tends to be a temporary 'slouching' posture, frequently seen in adolescents as they suddenly start to grow tall and 'shoot up'. However, it is still a cause of pain when held for longer periods. Correction involves tucking the chin in and lengthening

Flat-back posture

The flat-back posture shows a markedly reduced lumbar lordosis, and is commonly seen with those who sit for prolonged periods in their job. It is also common following back pain when a person has rested in bed. The individual is unable to move the spine correctly, and most of the structures around it are stiff and sore. Stiffness may limit either flexion or extension, and the spine becomes almost fixed in a flat-back position. Stretching can help to alleviate the pain from this condition as the lost flexibility is gradually regained. The stretches should feel slightly uncomfortable, because they are working on very tight structures; however, they should not give back pain. If they do, exercise should be carried out only under the supervision of a physiotherapist.

With the flat-back posture the spine is gradually stretched into extension (*see* table 5.2, (f)). When forward bending is also limited, flexion stretches may be performed using the hips for leverage (*see* table 5.2, (g)). In each case, the movement is gently encouraged rather than being vigorously forced.

Figure 5.18 Correcting the sway-back posture

Figure 5.19 Weak hip abductors altering the stepping gait: (a) normal muscle balance – abductors and adductors are the same length and strength; (b) imbalance – tight hip adductors inhibit (weaken) abductors. As the opposite foot is lifted from the ground, weak abductors fail to support the pelvis, allowing it to dip down.

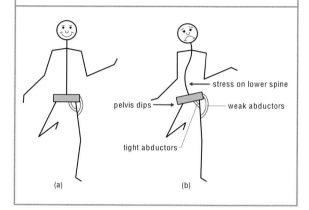

Key point: The flat-back is the classic sitting posture. With prolonged sitting, a person almost becomes 'chair shaped'. The lumbar curve is lost and the hips are tight and immobile.

Postural faults in the lower limbs

Postural faults in the foot and leg can be detrimental to knee health, and stretching can help to alleviate the faults. We have seen that imbalance between the various hip and lumbar spine muscles can alter the way in which the hip is extended when walking and running. A further imbalance pattern also exists between the hip abductor and adductor muscles. The adductors show a tendency to tighten, and this in turn inhibits the hip abductors. The abductor muscles are important stabilisers of the pelvis as we lift one leg from the ground, as in walking, stepping and running. As we lift the leg, the abductor muscles (especially gluteus medius) of the leg on the ground work hard to prevent the pelvis from dipping down. If these muscles are inhibited and weak, the pelvis dips, causing a sideways 'duck waddle' (*see* fig 5.19). This is most noticeable when performing step aerobics.

We saw in the PCS that when the hip extensors are weak, the hamstring muscles work by substitution, and in so doing they become tight. In the case of weak hip abductors, the tensor fascia lata muscle works instead. This muscle

Figure 5.20 Self-stretch of tight hip abductors: (a) hip hitching in standing; (b) abductor stretch after hip hitching

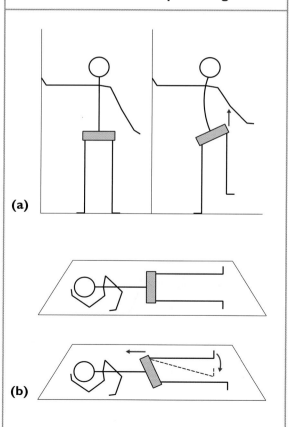

attaches to the ilio-tibial band (ITB), which travels down the side of the leg. The ITB, in turn, has a connection to the side of the knee with a small slip to the kneecap itself. Because the tensor fascia lata is having to work too hard to cover up for the weakened hip abductors, it tightens the ITB and pulls the kneecap outwards as weight is taken on one leg. This is a very common cause of a painful kneecap, often seen in sport.

> **Key point**: When we stand on one leg, the adductor muscles of the weight bearing leg 'hitch' the pelvis up, preventing it from sagging.

Correcting lower limb postural faults

The action now is clear. First, we must stretch the tight hip adductors. Then, if the condition has been present for some time, the ITB will be tight and will need to be stretched using the Ober test (see page 69). The test is performed, and the position of maximum stretch with the leg near the horizontal is held for 10–20 seconds. This should be practised daily with 5–8 repetitions.

To perform this technique without a partner requires good lateral stability of the pelvis. This may be assessed using a 'hip hitching', or 'leg shortening', exercise (*see* fig 5.20). In the side lying position, the upper leg is again abducted and slightly extended. From this position, the trunk side flexors are tightened by the hip hitching action. These muscles should remain tight as the upper leg is lowered, to prevent any lateral tilting of the pelvis. The stretch is felt over the outside of the hip.

Summary

- In a good posture, the body segments are aligned to minimise joint stress.
- A good posture requires minimal muscle work to maintain.
- Posture is assessed with reference to a 'plumb-line' from behind and the side.
- Local tests of muscle tightness are used to determine postural problems in specific parts of the body.
- Posture correction begins by enhancing core stability.
- A muscle imbalance correction programme is used to stretch tight muscle and strengthen/shorten lax muscle in order to realign body segments.

STRETCHING RESEARCH

6

In this chapter we will look at some of the research that has been conducted on the aspects of stretching covered in the rest of the book. Research is ongoing, so knowledge in this subject area is always increasing. Full details of recent research papers are listed in the reference section on p. 233.

> **Key point**: The length of the hamstrings is more important to pelvic control during forward bending than to static posture itself. When stretching the hamstrings, performing the exercise with an anterior pelvic tilt gives better results.

Stretching and posture

In a lordotic posture, the pelvis is anteriorly tilted and 'hangs on the hamstrings'. In this posture, the hamstrings are likely to be tight (increased tone), whereas in other postures their length is likely to be unrelated to pelvic tilt. Li et al. (1996) measured the importance of the length of the hamstrings. They took subjects with tight hamstrings who had a straight leg raise (SLR) of less than 70 degrees, and then applied a stretching programme. They found that the SLR improved and the motion of the pelvis in forward bending changed. Interestingly, the static postural alignment of the pelvis did not alter.

The importance of the pelvic tilt position when performing a hamstring stretch was addressed by Sullivan et al. (1992). They took 20 subjects with tight hamstrings and used static stretching and PNF techniques in either anterior or posterior pelvic tilt. Each subject performed ten minutes of stretching for four days per week over a two-week period. They found that the group who used a starting position of anterior pelvic tilt gained significantly greater hamstring flexibility.

Stretching and muscle stiffness

Halbertsma et al. (1996) looked at the load–deformation curve (*see* page 10) of stretched muscle. They took subjects with slightly short hamstrings (SLR less than 80 degrees) and applied ten minutes of static stretching for a single period. They found that the stress strain curves before and after exercise did not change, indicating that the stiffness of the muscle did not change in a single exercise bout; however, the range of motion increased.

To measure the effect of stretching on muscle stiffness, McNair and Stanley (1996) used oscillation of the calf muscles. In their experimental setup, subjects were seated with a weight on their knee and their foot on a rocker mechanism that allowed their heel to drop down into dorsiflexion, prestretching their calf muscles. Another weight was then dropped on the knee to rapidly stretch their muscles further. An accelerometer was connected to the weight holder resting on the leg to measure vertical movement and oscillation. The small movements that occurred were amplified 100 times, and an EMG recording demonstrated that no voluntary muscle contraction was occurring.

They found, first, that the elastic stiffness of the calf muscles reduced significantly after ten minutes jogging at 60 per cent of maximal heart rate; and that, second, the same effect was achieved after static stretching for five repetitions, holding each stretch for 30 seconds with a 30-second rest between each stretch.

Measuring the effect of tendon tap on the calf muscles was used to demonstrate the effect of stretching on muscle reflexes by Rosenbaum and Henning (1995). They showed improved muscle compliance after three minutes of static stretching of the calf muscles, and improved muscle force development and decreased EMG activity after a ten-minute warm-up run on a treadmill.

Magnusson et al. (1996) used the movement of an isokinetic dynamometer (*passive torque*) to measure the resistance of the hamstring muscles to stretch during passive knee extension. Passive torque is the force that a muscle exerts to 'push back' against the pressure of the machine. The subjects in the study performed a static hamstrings stretch, holding the stretch for 90 seconds. They performed five repetitions of this movement with a 30-second rest between each stretch. During the static stretch, passive torque reduced, indicating that the muscles were 'giving' a little. The stiffness of the muscles was also shown to reduce, but both measures returned to normal within one hour of testing.

> **Key point**: Static stretching has been shown to improve stretch tolerance, reduce muscle stiffness, and produce muscle changes which would tend to reduce the risk of injury.

Stretching as part of a warm-up

A warm-up will result in a number of physiological factors that may be of benefit to stretching.

Elevated temperature improves a person's ability to perform physical work in general as the critical level at which various metabolic chemical reactions occur is lower, so the reactions occur sooner (Bergh and Ekblom 1979). In addition, muscle contraction is more rapid and more forceful (Bergh 1980). The sensitivity of nerve receptors and the speed at which a nerve is able to transmit its impulse is quicker (Astrand and Rodahl 1986). The improvements in nerve conduction seen after a warm-up are particularly important for PNF stretching, for example, where reflex mechanisms are used to improve range of motion.

The stiffness (viscosity) of the synovial fluid limits a joint's range and ease of motion. The viscosity of the synovial fluid is reduced meaning that it offers less resistance, as its temperature rises during a warm-up (Astrand and Rodahl 1986). A greater force and length of stretch is required to tear muscle that has undergone a warm-up, due to the reduction in viscosity of the connective tissue within the muscle (Safran et al. 1988). LaBan (1962) showed a 1.5 per cent increase in the length of a stretched tendon following a temperature increase to 42.5°C, while Warren et al. (1971) demonstrated that a tendon heated to 45°C increased in length by 5.8 per cent and its force to failure was 58 per cent greater than that at a normal body temperature. Realistically, these extreme temperatures, compared to a normal body temperature of 38.9°C, can only be achieved through passive heating as used by a physiotherapist. However, they do demonstrate the importance of allowing tissue to warm before it is stretched.

Effects of temperature on pliability of body tissue

When a tissue is warmed, it takes a greater stretching force to tear it (Safran et al. 1988) due to a change in the resistance offered by the tissue, known as its 'viscoelastic' property. In the sixties and seventies, early research work demonstrated this effect quite clearly. Tendons could be stretched further before rupturing (LaBan 1962) and a 50–60 per cent greater force was needed before the tendon actually failed and tore (Warren et al 1971).

Ice also affects tissue pliability. When applied to the skin, ice causes a reduction in blood flow to the superficial tissues, but also causes a reddening of the skin (hyperaemia) as a protective effect. Following injury, the reduction of blood flow is used to slow the metabolic rate of the injured tissues and limit any damage caused by the injury. In terms of stretching however, the important feature of ice application is that it depresses muscle spindle activity, an important component of the stretch reflex (Halvorson 1990). Muscle spasm is reduced, and the muscle itself takes on a more relaxed state.

It must be remembered that the effect of ice is more likely reflex in nature, as the cold does not go very deeply into the body tissues. On the skin, the temperature reduction may be as much as 20°C after ice application for 20 minutes (Palmer and Knight 1996), but at a depth of only 1.7 cm the change in temperature reduces dramatically to 4°C (Zemke et al. 1998). In a joint, temperature reduction is unlikely, except for the superficial joints of the toes and fingers. Levy and Lintner (1997) found no significant temperature reduction in the shoulder (glenohumeral) joint, even after 90 minutes of ice application.

> **Key point**: When used as part of a warm up, stretching has beneficial effects on muscle, tendon, nerve and joint structures.

Does heat or ice improve stretching techniques?

Heat applied *before* static stretching does not result in a greater increase in range of motion from a hamstring stretch (Taylor et al. 1995).

When applied *together with* a static stretch, however, the story can be different, resulting in an increased range of motion at the hip, shoulder and shin (Shrier and Gossal, 2000). Ice applied in combination with a static stretch (cryostretch) is most effective when applied in the early stages of stretching (Lentell et al. 1992). However, the effect of cryostretch seems more appropriate to muscles in spasm through pain or injury.

On normal muscle, heat and cold do not seem to improve the effectiveness of stretching. Using an active knee extension (AKE) stretch, Taylor et al. (1995) examined static stretching alone and static stretching with either heat or cold; they found no difference between any of the groups. Cornelius et al. (1992) came to a similar conclusion concerning PNF stretching; they looked at static stretching and PNF stretching, with and without cold application, and found no significant differences between the groups.

> **Key point**: Both warming and cooling superficial tissues before stretching has some merit. Warmed tissue may be less likely to tear, and cold or ice may be useful where muscle spasm is present.

Injury prevention

Many athletes believe that warm-up and stretching will help to prevent injury and make them perform better. If stretching can offer less resistance to movement and increase range of motion, it is possible to see that a mechanism may exist to justify these claims. However, because there are many factors interrelated with injury and performance, these claims are as yet to be substantiated.

> **Key point**: Ice and heat do not seem to significantly improve the range of motion obtained by stretching, unless heat is applied at the same time as the stretch is performed.

The combination of warm-up and stretching has been shown by some authors to actually reduce the incidence of injury. Ekstrand et al. (1983) showed that a group of footballers performing a 20-minute warm-up, which included ten minutes of stretching, suffered only 75 per cent of the injuries that their colleagues, who did not perform the warm-up, did. Stretching as part of a rehabilitation programme has been also been shown to reduce the rate of injury recurrence to only 1 per cent following calf muscle injury (Millar 1976).

Stretching may also improve the efficiency of movement in certain circumstances. In one study (Godges et al. 1989), the economy of running gait was shown to improve at both moderate and high exercise intensities through increases in hip range of motion thanks to stretching exercises. Other studies, however, have shown the reverse. Gleim et al. (1990) showed that 'tighter' subjects were significantly more economical as fast walkers and joggers than more flexible subjects. The tighter subjects also demonstrated better oxygen consumption values on treadmill activities.

Research by Krivickas and Feinberg (1996) tested 200 college athletes and found that the risk of injury decreased as flexibility improved. These authors showed a 15 per cent increased risk of injury for those who were less flexible and a 20 per cent reduced risk for those who were more flexible. However, the opposite was found by Askling et al. (2002) when looking at hamstring flexibility in ballet dancers; they showed that stretching could give rise to injury in the upper portion of the hamstrings. In a study of over 1,500 army recruits over a 12-week period, Pope et al. (2000) found 158 injuries in those who stretched and 175 in those who did not, but, when analysed statistically, the results showed no significant difference between the stretching and non-stretching (control) group.

Some authors have investigated the stretching studies themselves to determine the quality of the research involved. A study by two Australian physiotherapists (Herbert and Gabriel 2002) summarised the information gained from five scientific studies, and concluded that there was no evidence that stretching – either before or after exercise – protects against muscle soreness or injury. In a later study, two UK-based osteopaths (Weldon and Hill 2003) conducted a review of seven papers and decided that no definitive conclusions could be made concerning the value of stretching due to the poor quality of the available studies. However, a systematic review by Fradkin et al (2006) looked at papers (all high quality randomised controlled trials) between 1966–2005 and concluded that 'the weight of evidence is in favour of decreased risk of injury'.

The jury is certainly still out on this one. Athletes and coaches often believe that stretching is beneficial in some way as regards injury prevention, but the research is yet to determine first, if any benefit exists, and second, how any such benefit could be obtained. Based on the current research, the recommendation must be that, before physical exertion of any type, an active warm up to increase both tissue and joint temperature is probably better than simply static stretching alone. In addition, a specific warm-up to match the movement patterns of the sport to be undertaken is likely to optimally prepare the athlete from the point of view of motor control (Shrier 2000, Shrier and Gossal 2000).

Key point: Before sport, use an active warm up to increase both tissue and joint temperature, and a specific warm up to match the movement patterns of the sport.

If stretching does prevent injury, how is this achieved? This is a problem addressed by a team from Ghent University in Belgium (Witvrouw et al 2004) who considered the type of activity to be one of the most important factors in determining whether stretching was effective at preventing injuries or not. Exercises which require bouncing and jumping activities (plyometrics, *see* page 000) require the muscle-tendon unit to be springy and compliant, in other words less 'stiff'. This, as we have seen, is a feature which stretching can achieve. If athletes performing these tasks have a stiffer muscle-tendon unit the demands placed on it by high intensity exercise may exceed the tissue capacity, causing injury. In those athletes who use only low intensity exercise (jogging for example) there may be no advantage to having a muscle-tendon unit which is less stiff, and so injury prevention is not likely to be seen here.

> **Key point**: Long term stretching reduces stiffness in the muscle-tendon unit which may be protective in some power sports.

Muscle reflexes and stretching

The effects of stretching on muscle reflexes are often investigated by measuring the excitability of a muscle. To do this, a *Hoffmann reflex* (H reflex) is used. We saw that, when a muscle is stretched rapidly, it responds by evoking a stretch reflex (*see* page 29). The Hoffman reflex is similar, except that it is an artificial reflex. If a muscle, usually the soleus in the calf, is electrically stimulated with a single shock, a muscle twitch results and is seen on an EMG machine. The strength of this muscle twitch (H reflex) is recorded as the height of the EMG signal graph. If a group of motor nerve cells (motor neuron pool) is more active (excitable), the H reflex will be stronger because more motor nerves are involved in the contraction.

A number of factors will influence the excitability of the motor neuron pool. For example, if a subject clenches their teeth by biting hard, the H reflex is stronger, demonstrating that the motor nerves to all muscle will be excited. Although there is no logical connection from the jaw to the calf, there is a functional relationship that is important to stretching. When we grip any muscle tightly, in this case the jaw, neural signals are sent not just to the muscle concerned, but along the spinal cord as well. This has the effect of 'setting' the muscles and bracing our posture to create stability. This effect, known as the *Jendrassik manoeuvre*, is important, because if we are trying to stretch a muscle using PNF techniques, we want that muscle to relax and offer less resistance to the stretching force. If we place a subject in a starting position where they are unbalanced and gripping on to something, or where they feel insecure, the increased tone that results will have a knock-on effect to the tone of the muscle we are stretching, even though that muscle may be some distance away.

Research into the response of muscle to PNF stretching has used the H reflex to assess muscle excitability after isometric contraction using the contract–relax method (*see* page 60). Moore and Kukulka (1991) showed the H reflex to be suppressed after isometric contraction. The excitability of the motor nerve and of the stretch reflex mechanism itself appears to decrease following isometric contractions, and this decreased level lasts for about ten seconds, whether or not the muscle was contracted for one second or 30 seconds. This gives a 10-second 'window' in which to apply the stretch.

Looking at the EMG trace to judge the efficiency of the stretch reflex, Nicol et al. (1996) used a maximum vertical depth jump. They found that both reflex activity and muscle biochemistry changed considerably: creatine kinase activity increased, showing micro-damage to the muscle fibres (as occurs with eccentric exercise);

the stretch reflex sensitivity was reduced completely by the second day after exhaustive exercise; and recovery was not fully complete until four days after the exercise.

Key point: Exhaustive exercise, especially that which is likely to cause muscle damage, such as eccentric actions, reduces the sensitivity of the stretch reflex and may remove some of its protective function. This makes injury more likely.

Types of stretching

Several researchers have asked the question, 'Which is the best way to stretch?' Static stretching seems to be as effective as ballistic stretching, except that ballistic stretching creates a considerable amount of muscle soreness (Etnyre and Abraham 1986). PNF techniques provide greater improvements in range of motion than either static or ballistic methods (Enoka 1994).

Webright et al. (1997) compared static stretching with active stretching. They took 40 subjects through a stretching programme in a sitting position. Initially, subjects were unable to lock their knee (minimum of 15 degrees short of full extension) when sitting with the femur at 90 degrees and statically stretching the hamstrings. One group practiced static stretching (a single repetition held for 30 seconds), while the other practiced slow (non-ballistic) active knee extension (30 repetitions, each taking one second). Each group performed two bouts of stretching daily for six weeks. The results showed that both groups developed an equal amount of flexibility, with the subjects changing from 15 degrees short of full extension to 8–10 degrees short of full extension. Importantly, this programme demonstrated significant increases in flexibility in just six weeks through a short (30-second) stretching programme performed daily.

Key point: PNF stretching gives superior gains in range of motion, and even brief stretching programmes (of any type) are effective, providing they are practised regularly.

Stretches – how long and how many?

The exact amount of time needed to effectively stretch has been the subject of many studies. Bandy and Irion (1994) used knee extension to test static stretch timing. They chose 47 subjects with limited knee extension and subjected them to 15-, 30-, or 60-second static stretches. Each group stretched for five days a week over a period of six weeks. Their results showed that both the 30- and 60-second stretches were more effective than the 15-second stretch, but, importantly, the 60-second stretch gave no greater gains than the 30-second one. The conclusion they made was that there is no advantage in holding a stretch for 60 seconds; 30 seconds seems to be an adequate period to hold a static stretch.

Because the effects of stretching are cumulative (see page 50), a number of repetitions are normally performed. Taylor et al. (1990) found that the greatest effects of stretch to the muscle and tendon occurred during the first four stretches, with a greater number of repetitions failing to produce greater improvements. In this case, more did not seem to be better!

Key point: Optimal stretching timing is 4–5 repetitions, holding each repetition for 30 seconds.

Limiting factors in range of movement

Two factors limit the possible range of motion available at a joint: contractile and non-contractile structures. The degree of limitation presented by the various tissues varies between joints. In the spine, Adams et al. (1980) looked at cadavers and found that the vertebral disc limits flexion and extension movements by 29 per cent, while the supraspinous and interspinous ligaments limit the same movement by 19 per cent. The facet joint capsules have the greatest limitation to movement, at 39 per cent. For the metacarpophalangeal joints, the capsule limits movement by 47 per cent, muscle by 41 per cent, tendons by 10 per cent and skin by 2 per cent (Johns and Wright 1992).

When muscles are relaxed, the improvement in range of motion with each successive stretch will increase. Taylor et al. (1990) used the extensor digitorum longus muscle in the leg, stretched it by a set amount and held the stretch for 30 seconds. Each bout of stretches consisted of 10 repetitions. Two outcomes emerged from this research: first, to produce the same resistance force, the muscle had to be stretched further by 3.5 per cent; and, second, when the muscle was stretched to a pre-set length, the load required to do this gradually reduced. The conclusion is that, over time, the passive resistance offered by muscle to a stretch reduces. Thus static or PNF stretching seems to be more effective than ballistic stretching. In addition, each stretch should be held and the individual stretches repeated for a set of ten or more repetitions.

> **Key point**: Both contractile (muscle) and non-contractile (other tissue) factors limit range of motion and provide resistance to movement. With prolonged stretching, the passive resistance produced by a muscle is reduced.

Does stretching alter muscle power output?

Anyone will recognise that after a hard stretching session the muscles feel shaky and slightly weak. This feeling actually identifies a recognised physiological effect, that of a reduction in strength output following intense stretching. Following hip and knee stretching, Kokkonen et al. (1998) tested subjects with a one repetition maximum (1RM) lift. (1RM, or '1 repetition maximum', is the maximum amount of weight that can be lifted in a single repetition.) The subjects' lifting ability was reduced by 7–8 per cent following static stretching.

Using a footplate to stretch and measure strength output from the deep calf (soleus) muscle, Fowles et al. (2000) used 13 maximal passive stretches over a 30-minute period, holding each stretch for over two minutes. Again, they measured maximal muscle contraction and found that strength in the stretching group reduced by 28 per cent immediately after stretching, reducing to 12 per cent after 30 minutes and 9 per cent after 60 minutes. Using a leg extension exercise, Behm et al. (2001) used 20 minutes of static stretching, with each repetition held for 45 seconds. These authors found a 12 per cent reduction in maximal leg strength, confirming the results of the previous studies. A number of mechanisms may be responsible for this stretch-induced decline in strength output.

Electrical monitoring of muscle activity (EMG) has revealed a 20 per cent decline in quadriceps activity after stretching (Behm et al. 2001). Stimulating the muscle electrically (a method called interpolated twitch or IT) has also shown decreases in muscle activation of up to 13 per cent (Fowles et al. 2000). We have seen that a variety of muscle reflexes are important to stretching, and it seems that these may contribute to the strength changes. Changes in the stretch reflex and golgi tendon organs have both been proposed as other contributing factors.

Finally, after intense eccentric muscle contraction, there is microscopic damage within the muscle, leading to an increase in a chemical called creatine kinase (CK). Levels of this same chemical are raised by over 60 per cent following intense stretching (Smith et al. 1993), so it seems that muscle damage may also result from intense stretching.

> **Key point**: Intense stretching prior to performance is not recommended, as it will likely result in reduced power output from the muscle. Intense stretching should be an entirely separate part of a training programme.

So, we can see that prior stretching (stretching before performance) can be detrimental to muscle power output. But, what about strength endurance – that is performing multiple reps rather than a single rep? This is a question answered by Nelson et al (2005) from Louisiana State University. They had athletes perform strength endurance activities at 60 per cent bodyweight and at 40 per cent bodyweight, with and without prior stretching. Strength endurance was reduced by 24 per cent at 60 per cent bodyweight exercise and by 9 per cent at 40 per cent bodyweight. Both results were statistically significant, and the larger reduction reflects the greater effect of prior stretching on heavier power based exercise.

Does stretching improve performance?

Shrier, a researcher from Quebec, Canada, looked at whether stretching can actually improve performance (Shrier 2004). Rather than testing individual athletes, Shrier looked at 23 articles which examined the effects of acute stretching (the effect immediately after a stretch has been performed), and nine articles looking at the effects of regular stretching. Analysis of these articles showed that there was no improvement of isometric force, isokinetic torque (individual muscle measures) or jumping height (whole body measure) after acute stretching. Of the nine papers which looked at the long term effect of stretching seven papers actually demonstrated improvements in force, jump height and speed.

> **Key point**: Regular stretching can improve muscle power, but short term stretching does not.

Summary

- The angle of pelvic tilt is important for the application of stretches around the hip, especially for the hamstrings.
- Stretching reduces the 'stiffness' in a muscle in much the same way as a warm-up does. Over time, this may have a protective effect on the muscle-tendon unit in power based activities.
- Tendon, ligaments, nerves and the joint capsule will also limit range of motion at a joint.
- Ice may be used to reduce muscle spasm prior to stretching.
- Following intense stretching, the power output of a muscle can be reduced.
- Combining heat with stretching will give better results than warming prior to stretching.
- Muscle reflexes are important to the stretching process.
- A 30-second static stretch is most effective, and four or five repetitions only should be applied.
- Intense stretching immediately before competitive sport is not recommended.

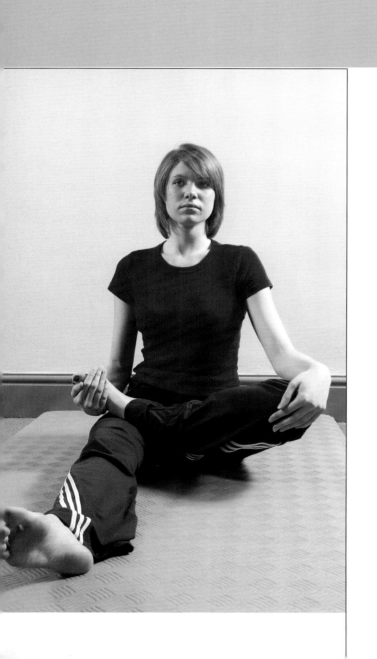

PART **TWO**

THE EXERCISES

BEGINNER STRETCHES

7

Introduction to the stretching exercises

In this chapter we begin to look at a variety of stretching exercises. The list is by no means exhaustive, but it includes the most useful exercises for sport. The exercises are loosely grouped into sections, each under a separate chapter number. The beginner, intermediate and advanced stretch groupings take into account the complexity of the movement, and the difficulty of performing the exercises with good alignment. However, any movement may become an advanced stretch simply by pressing into a greater range of motion. Within each of these chapters the order of the exercises is based on three main areas of the body: lower limbs, trunk and upper limbs, respectively. Tables 7.1(a), 7.1(b) and 7.1(c) provide details of the muscles stretched for each exercise movement for each of these areas of the body. There are also chapters showing stretches for the nerves (neural stretches), linked tissues (fascial stretches), partner stretches and stretches that a therapist or personal trainer may apply to a client.

Before performing any of the movements, make sure that you are thoroughly warmed up; you should be sweating lightly and wrapped in loose-fitting clothing to maintain body-heat. All exercises should be performed slowly, encouraging, rather than forcing, the

action. The stretch should be placed on the muscle when exhaling, and the final position held for 20–30 seconds, while breathing normally. You should feel a comfortable stretch, but no pain.

Starting position and instructions refer to the right-hand side of the body, but can be applied to the left-hand side just as easily. 'Lie on the floor' will always refer to lying on your back, unless otherwise stated.

Variations of exercises are included because these prevent you from getting stale. In addition, two or three exercises designed to stretch exactly the same muscles will each stress the body in slightly different ways. These different stresses reduce the likelihood of developing overuse injuries. You will have preferences for certain exercises, and some will suit you more than others, depending on your body-size and make-up. This is fine, and serves to individualise your stretching programme.

Points to note are important because these are sometimes points to note concerned with safety factors and injury prevention. You may like to make a note of any points you find relevant to your own training style after reading this section on an exercise.

The following are also useful references: figure 1.14 Axes and planes (*see* page 13), figure 1.15 Anatomical terminology (*see* page 14), and table 4.5 Starting positions (*see* page 61).

Table 7.1(a)	Upper limb
Joint movement	**Muscles stretched**
Shoulder protraction	Rhomboid major; rhomboid minor; trapezius
Shoulder retraction	Serratus anterior; pectoralis minor
Shoulder depression	Trapezius (upper fibres), levator scapulae
Shoulder adduction	Suprasinatus, deltoid
Shoulder extension	Pectoralis major, deltoid (anterior fibres), biceps brachii (long head), coracobrachialis
Shoulder flexion	Latissimus dorsi, teres major, pectoralis major, deltoid (posterior fibres), triceps (long head)
Shoulder abduction	Coracobrachialis, pectoralis major, latissimus dorsi, teres major
Shoulder lateral rotation	Subscapularis, teres major, latissimus dorsi, pectoralis major, deltoid (anterior fibres)
Shoulder medial rotation	Teres minor, infraspinatus, deltoid (posterior fibres)
Elbow extension	Biceps brachii, brachialis, brachioradialis, pronator teres
Elbow flexion	Triceps brachii, anconeus
Forearm supination	Pronator teres, pronator quadratus, brachiordialis
Wrist extension	Flexor carpi ulnaris, flexor carpi radialis, Palmaris longus, flexor digitorum superficialis, flexor digitorum profundus, flexor pollicis longus
Wrist flexion	Extensor carpi radialis longus, extensor, carpi radialis brevis, extensor carpi ulnaris, extensor digitorum, extensor indicis, extensor digiti minimi, extensor pollicis longus, extensor pollicis brevis

Table 7.1(b)	Trunk
Joint movement	**Muscles served**
Extension	Rectus abdominis, external oblique, internal oblique, psoas minor, psoas major
Rotation	Multifidus, rotatores, semispinalis, internal oblique, external oblique
Lateral flexion	Quadratus lumborum, intertransversarii, external oblique, internal oblique, rectus abdominis, erector spinae, multifidus
Flexion	Quadratus lumborum, multifidus, semispinalis, erector spinae, interspinales

Table 7.1(c)	Lower limb
Joint movement	**Muscle stretched**
Hip flexion	Gluteus maximus, hamstrings (semiendinosus, semimembranosus, biceps femoris)
Hip adduction	Gluteus maximus, gluteus medius, gluteus minimus, tensor fascia lata
Hip abduction	Adductor magnus, adductor longus, adductor brevis, gracilis, pectineus
Hip extension	Psoas major, iliacus, rectus femoris, Sartorius, pectineus
Hip lateral (outward) rotation	Anterior part of gluteus medius, anterior part of gluteus minimus, tensor fascia lata, psoas major, iliacus
Hip medial (inward) rotation	Gluteus maximus, piriformis, obturator internus, gemellus superior, gemellus inferior, quadratus femoris, obturator externus
Knee joint extension	Hamstrings (semitendinosus, semimembranosus, biceps femoris), gastrocnemius, gracilis, Sartorius
Knee joint flexion	Quadriceps femoris (rectus femoris, vastus lateralis, vastus intermedius, vastus medialis), tensor fascia lata
Ankle joint dorsiflexion	Gastrocnemius, soleus, plantaris, peroneus longus, tibialis posterior, flexor digitorum longus, flexor hallucis longus
Ankle joint plantarflexion	Tibialis anterior, extensor digitorum longus, extensor hallucis longus, peroneus tertius

Exercise 1	**Hip adductors – long sitting**

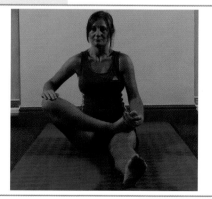

Starting position and instructions

Sit on the floor with both legs straight. Flex your right leg, placing your foot on your left thigh above the knee. Support the foot with your left hand, and press down on the knee with your right hand. Lengthen your spine and maintain spinal alignment throughout the movement.

Variations

Start by sitting with your back flat against a wall and a rolled towel placed in the small of your back (lumbar area) to maintain spinal alignment. You can sit on a wedge to anteriorly tilt the pelvis. If your knee is too stiff to bend so that your foot rests on your thigh, rest your foot just below the knee, on the shin.

Points to note

Most individuals are asymmetrical and will find that one leg is more flexible than the other. There is a tendency with this exercise for those who have reduced flexibility of the adductors to tilt the body towards the bent knee, lifting the pelvis and buttock (ischial) from the floor. This gives an apparent increase in flexibility as the knee can be lowered further, but there is no greater stretch placed on the adductors.

Exercise 2	Gluteal stretch – lying

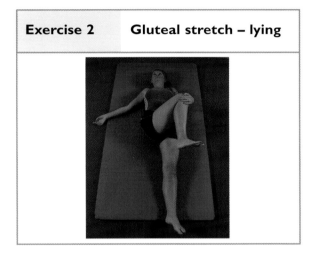

Starting position and instructions

Lie on the floor with the left leg straight. Flex the right knee and pull it upwards and across towards the left shoulder.

Variations

Pulling the knee across the body rather than towards the shoulder will vary the emphasis of the stretch.

Points to note

This exercise also places stress on the pelvis, so it is inappropriate after pregnancy. Also, the combination of extreme hip flexion and adduction makes the exercise dangerous to those who have had a hip replacement operation.

Exercise 3	Hamstrings stretch – long sitting

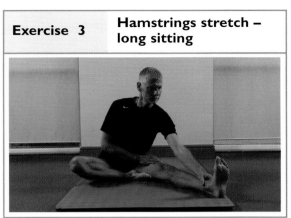

Starting position and instructions

Sit with your right leg straight and your left leg comfortably bent. Reach forwards with the right hand to grip the sole of your right foot. Press your left hand on your right knee to maintain knee extension. Maintain spinal alignment, gently curving throughout the whole spine.

Variations

Place both hands on the right knee, lengthen your spine and hinge only from the hip avoiding spinal flexion. Alternatively, loop a belt or towel under your foot and pull on the belt rather than on the foot directly. Placing the belt under the ball of the foot and toes rather than the heel will cause an additional stretch on the tissue that forms the sole of the foot (plantarfascia).

Points to note

Individuals who are hyperflexible in the thoracic spine may place excessive stress on this area. To avoid this, retract the shoulders, expand the chest and maintain this position throughout the exercise. If you find you are still unable to maintain your spinal alignment, reverse the order of the exercise to change the emphasis. Begin with your knee unlocked (slightly bent) and reach forward with a straight spine. Once in the stretched position, attempt to straighten the leg.

Exercise 4	Hamstrings – active knee extension

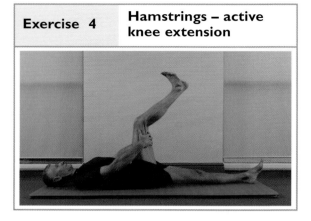

Exercise 5	Knee extension – with towel

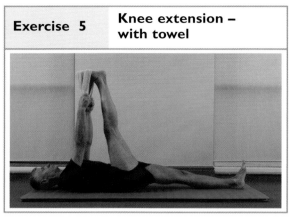

Starting position and instructions

Lie on the floor with the left leg straight and flex the right knee and hip to 90 degrees. Grip your hands behind the right knee and actively straighten the leg using your quadriceps muscles. The knee should remain directly above the hip.

Variations

Place your hand on the front of the leg and actively push your leg on to your hand using the power of your hip flexors; at the same time, extend your knee. This will cause the hamstring muscles to further relax through reflex action.

Points to note

Pulling the toes towards you and flexing your neck will throw stress on to the neural tissues and sciatic nerve and away from the hamstrings (*see* page 165).

Starting position and instructions

Lie on the floor with the left leg straight and flex the right knee and hip to 90 degrees. Hook a folded towel around your right foot, holding one end of the towel in each hand. Rest your upper arms on the mat and attempt to straighten your leg by pushing your foot into the towel. Do not allow your arms to straighten, and keep the hip, knee and foot in a straight line.

Variations

Instead of a towel, use an exercise band. Make sure that the band is in the centre of the foot rather than on the toes to guard against slipping.

Points to note

Fastening the towel over your toes will pull the toes towards you. Combining this movement with flexion of the neck will throw stress on to the neural tissues and sciatic nerve and away from the hamstrings (*see* page 165).

Exercise 6	Hamstrings stretch – supported by door frame

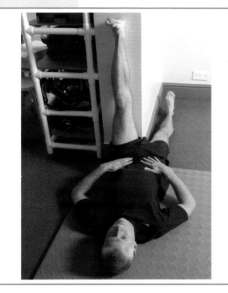

Exercise 7	Rectus femoris stretch – standing

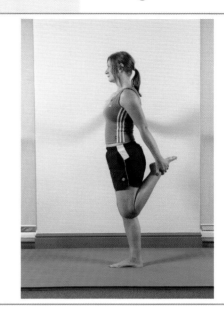

Starting position and instructions

Start by lying on the floor in a doorway. Your hips should be level with the doorframe. Bend your left leg and place your left foot on the upright of the frame, keeping your right leg straight on the ground. Straighten your left leg, sliding your left heel up the doorframe as you do so.

Variations

Moving your whole body forwards or backwards so that the door frame is at waist or knee level will cause a greater or lesser amount of hip flexion and change the intensity of the exercise.

Points to note

Make sure that your heel stays on the door frame to take the weight of your leg. If you find that your foot does not slide readily, keep your sock on to increase slip.

Starting position and instructions

Stand side-on to a wall with your left hand supporting your body-weight. Flex your right leg and grip your ankle with your knee flexed. Pull your right hip back into extension, while maintaining correct spinal alignment.

Variations

Loop a towel around your ankle to reduce the amount of knee flexion and to allow you to pull in to further hip extension, which will emphasise the upper portion of the muscle.

Points to note

This exercise also stretches the femoral nerve (*see* page 173). A sensation of burning or tingling (pins and needles) over the front of the thigh suggests that this nerve may be tight or possibly trapped, requiring physiotherapy management,

Exercise 8	Calf stretch – wall lean

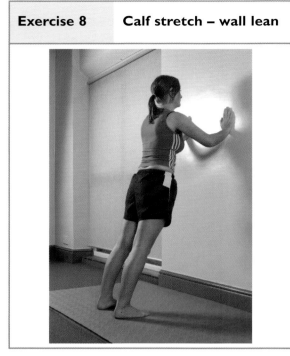

Exercise 9	Calf lunge

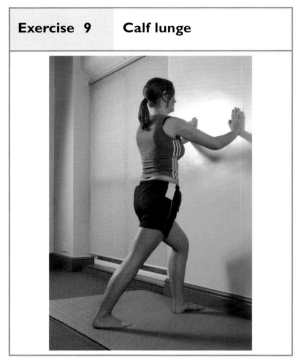

Starting position and instructions

Stand facing a wall with both feet together, arms straight and hands on the wall. Keeping your legs straight, bend your arms to lower your trunk towards the wall.

Variations

Walking towards or away from the wall will change the emphasis of the exercise.

Points to note

Asymmetry is common in this area, so you may find that one arm can bend more than the other. This movement stretches the superficial calf muscle, the gastrocnemius .

Starting position and instructions

Begin by facing a wall in a half-lunge position with your right foot forward. Place your hands on the wall and bend your arms to lower your body-weight forwards, pressing your right foot into dorsiflexion.

Variations

Altering the angle of the foot away from the perpendicular will change the emphasis on the calf muscle.

Points to note

The heel must remain on the floor throughout the movement. As the knee is bent in this movement, the stretch on the superficial calf muscle (gastrocnemius) is reduced and that on the deep calf muscle (soleus) increased.

Exercise 10	Lower back flexion – lying

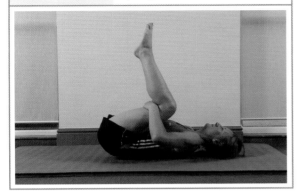

Exercise 11	Whole back flexion – sitting

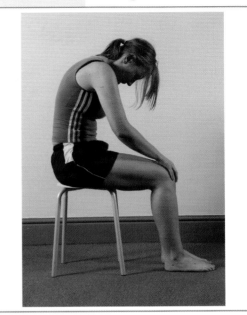

Starting position and instructions

Lie on the floor, drawing your knees up to your chest. Grip your knees and pull them into your chest and up towards your shoulders, creating a rocking position in your lower spine. This movement stretches the erector spinae.

Variations

This movement can be combined with rotation or lateral flexion to alter the stress on your spine.

Points to note

The movement is one of pulling your knees towards your shoulders rather than pulling your knees in towards your chest.

Starting position and instructions

Begin by sitting on a stool or firm chair with your hips slightly above your knees and your feet hip width apart. Place your hands on your thighs to take some of the weight of your trunk throughout the movement. Start the movement by bending your neck and pulling your chin down to your chest. Continue the action by flexing your thoracic spine, aiming your nose towards your umbilicus, and finally allow the lumbar spine to bend as though bringing your head between your knees. Pause in the lower position and then straighten your spine section by section until you are sitting upright again.

Variations

You can emphasise different sections of your spine with this movement. Beginning with neck flexion initiates movement at the upper thoracic spine, while keeping the neck in line with the rest of the spine throws the stretch to the mid- and lower thoracic spine. As you bend forwards, tucking the tail under (posterior pelvic tilt) throws the emphasis lower down the lumbar spine.

Points to note

Make sure that you begin the exercise by taking most of your upper body weight through your hands. As you become more confident with the movement, you can change the exercise into more of a controlled strength action by releasing the arms and allowing them to hang at the sides of the knees. In this way, you control the action using an eccentric (muscle lengthening) action of the spinal extensors going down and a concentric (muscle shortening) action as you come back up.

The action should feel as though your spine is a column of bricks; as you bend, you are moving one brick at a time, un-stacking and then stacking the vertebrae back up again.

Exercise 12	Thoracic spine – kneeling

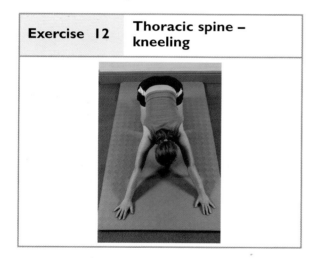

Starting position and instructions

Kneeling on all fours, sit back on your ankles, keeping your hands fixed. Feel the stretch in the latissimus dorsi muscle and thoracolumbar fascia and the thoracic spine.

Variations

Placing one knee slightly forwards of the other will impart some lateral flexion on your spine.

Points to note

This position may be held for 30–120 seconds to gain full benefit of the stretch on your spine.

Exercise 13	Thoracic spine – sitting

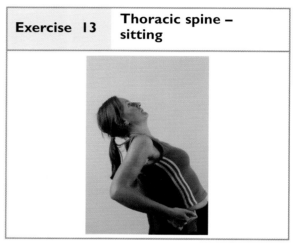

Starting position and instructions

Begin by sitting on a high backed chair with a towel folded over the top of the chair-back for padding. Sit right back in the chair so that your buttocks actually contact the chair back. Extend your thoracic spine over the back of the chair using the padded upper edge as a pivot point. Draw your elbows and upper arms backwards to supply force for the stretch.

Variations

The exact point at which the stretch is felt will depend on the contact point between the upper edge of the chair-back and the thoracic spine. Shuttling up and down to place the chair edge higher or lower on the spine will vary the emphasis of the stretch.

Points to note

As you extend the thoracic spine backwards, make sure that your hips do not simply slide forwards, as this will release part of the stretch, reducing its effectiveness. As you extend the thoracic spine, the ribcage will be expanded, so breath in as you stretch and out as you release it.

Exercise 14	Shoulder rotation

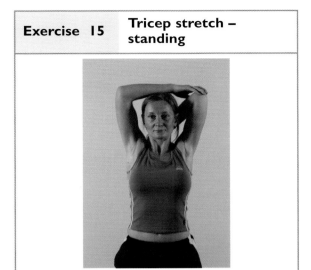

Exercise 15	Tricep stretch – standing

Starting position and instructions

Kneel and internally rotate and extend the shoulders to place your hands behind you on the small of your back. Draw your elbows back and together to stretch the external rotators and flexors of the shoulder (teres minor, supraspinatus, infraspinatus, deltoid and long head of the biceps muscles).

Variations

Moving the hands up towards the shoulders, or down towards the knees, will vary the site the of stretch.

Points to note

Optimal spinal alignment must be maintained throughout this exercise. The lumbar spine must not be hyperextended.

Starting position and instructions

Stand with your feet hip width apart. Reach overhead with your right arm and bend the elbow so that your right hand touches behind your right shoulder. Reach up with your left hand and grip your right elbow, pressing the right arm towards the vertical.

Variations

Bending the elbow less far (to 90 degrees rather than to full extension) will take some of the stretch away from the lower portion of the triceps and throw proportionally more stretch onto the upper portion. This is because the triceps is a two-joint (biarticular) muscle with actions over both the shoulder and the elbow.

Points to note

If you find that you have a tendency to lean backwards as you press your elbow overhead, perform the exercise sitting on a gym bench to aid the maintenance of spinal alignment.

INTERMEDIATE STRETCHES

Exercise 16	Calf and Achilles – prolonged stretch

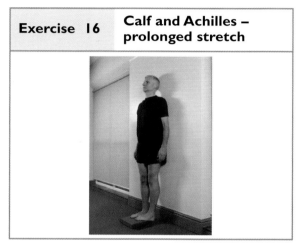

Starting position and instructions

Stand with your back against a wall and your feet about 10 cm in front of your bodyline. Place your toes and forefeet on a small (2 cm high) block or book and allow your heels to rest on the floor. Rest your body against the wall and maintain the position for 5–10 minutes.

Variations

Choosing a thicker block increases the stretch, while a thinner one reduces it. In each case, it is important that the heel rests on the floor throughout the exercise.

Points to note

This exercise offers a prolonged low-level stretch on the calf and Achilles. Because the heel rests on the floor, the calf muscles are able to relax instead of having to hold the position through an eccentric contraction. The combination of muscle relaxation and the length of time the stretch is held for makes this movement suitable for stretching after injury where swelling has built up and clotted to form tough scar tissue within the muscle or tendon.

Exercise 17	Anterior tibials

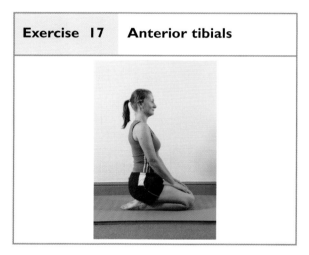

Starting position and instructions

Kneel on the floor and then sit back on your ankles, pressing the front of the ankles to the floor.

Variations

Place a folded towel beneath your toes to press them into flexion and increase the stretch on the toe extensors.

Points to note

This exercise places considerable stress on the knees. People with knee pain should perform the exercise leaning on a stool to support their bodyweight through.

Exercise 18	Hip flexors – Thomas test position

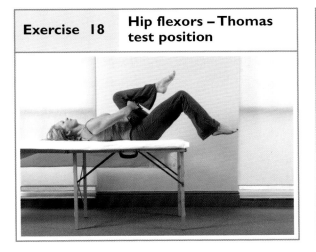

Exercise 19	Hip flexors – half-lunge position

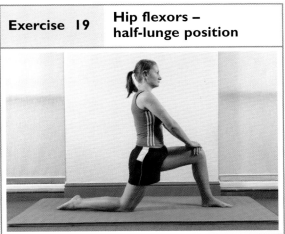

Starting position and instructions

Lie on a bench with your left leg over the bench end. Flex your right hip and knee and pull your knee towards your chest.

Variations

Start with both knees bent and the feet flat on the bench. Pull one knee to the chest and then lower the opposite leg.

Points to note

This is a basic clinical test of hip flexor tightness in the iliopsoas and rectus femoris of the lower leg: increasing the flexion at the knee emphasises the rectus femoris; reducing the knee flexion (straightening the leg) emphasises the iliopsoas.

Starting position and instructions

Kneel on your left leg with your right leg straight out in front of you and tighten your abdominal muscles to stabilise your trunk. Press your right leg forwards, forcing your left hip into extension.

Variations

Support your weight with one hand on a stool, or place your right forearm along the length of your right thigh. If you find yourself tending to lose spinal alignment, reach your left arm overhead as though trying to touch the ceiling; lengthening the entire body will help to emphasise good spinal alignment.

Points to note

Altering the degree of hip rotation will change the emphasis on the hip flexors. Relaxing the abdominal muscles and allowing the pelvis to tilt forwards will give the impression of a greater range of motion at the hip, but will actually stress the lumbar spine.

Exercise 20	Bilateral hip adductors – sitting

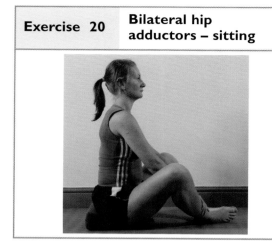

Exercise 21	Short adductor wall stretch

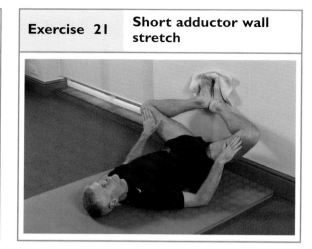

Starting position and instructions

Sit on the floor and place the soles of your feet together. Grip your feet and press down on your knees or thighs using your elbows. Maintain spinal alignment and try to lengthen your spine, reaching your head towards the ceiling as you press down with your elbows. Do not allow your pelvis to tilt backwards.

Variations

Sit on a wedge so that your pelvis is tilted forwards and your spine maintains its lumbar lordosis.

Points to note

Because the adductor muscles are attached to the pubic bone there is a tendency with this exercise to tilt the pelvis backwards and bring the pubic bone forwards, releasing the stretch from the muscle. When this is done the knee will lower further, but there is no greater stretch placed on the adductors. Maintaining the lumbar lordosis and the neutral pelvic position is therefore essential.

Starting position and instructions

Lie on the floor with your legs straight up and your buttocks close to the wall. Bend your knees and place the soles of your feet together with the sides of your feet resting on the wall itself. Place your hands over your knees and gently press your knees down towards the wall.

Variations

You may keep one leg straight, and place the foot of your bend knee on the straight leg thigh mimicking the position of exercise 1.

Points to note

This exercise is similar to exercise 20, but with the whole body rotated through 90 degrees. Now, instead of the legs being supported on the floor allowing the back to bend, the back is kept straight throughout the movement. If your find your arms are not long enough to reach to your knees without flexing your spine, use two small blocks (yoga bricks) placed on your thighs to 'lengthen your arms'.

Exercise 22	Hip adductors – wide splits

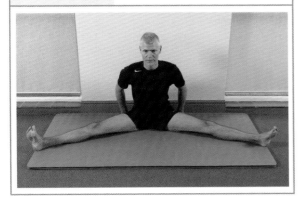

Exercise 23	Hip adductors – wall support

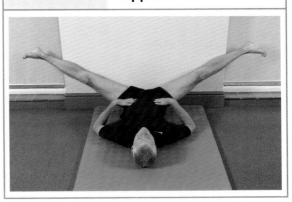

Starting position and instructions

Sit on a gym ball with your knees and hips bent to 90 degrees. Your feet should be wider than shoulder width apart and flat on the floor. Walk your feet forwards so that the gym ball rolls under your back and stop when it lies between your shoulder blades. Straighten your arms and reach over your head and back towards the floor, allowing your hips to drop down towards the floor at the same time.

Variations

By adjusting the position of the gym ball, you can determine which area of your spine receives the greatest stretch.

Points to note

This is an extreme stretch, but is quite comfortable to hold as the whole of the spine is supported. If you find the stretch too difficult, deflate the gym ball slightly so that it is flatter and more squashy. The flatter contour of the ball will reduce the intensity of the stretch.

Starting position and instructions

Lie on the floor with your legs straight up in the air and your buttocks close to a wall. Rest your legs against the wall and allow them to lower slowly out to the sides and downwards into hip abduction. Hold this position for 20–30 seconds and then bring the legs back up again by 20–30 cm (resisted adduction), before again allowing them to lower.

Variations

Lifting the legs against their own weight provides resistance for contract–relax (CR) stretching. This can be increased by having your training partner resist the adduction movement for you by pressing down on your legs.

Points to note

Although this is a stretching exercise, the legs are lowered by an eccentric contraction of the hip adductor muscles and then held in place by an isometric contraction of the same muscles. As the hip adductors relax, movement is increased. The exercise therefore serves to aid adductor muscle relaxation, reducing muscle tone.

Exercise 24	Hamstrings and spine – sit and reach position

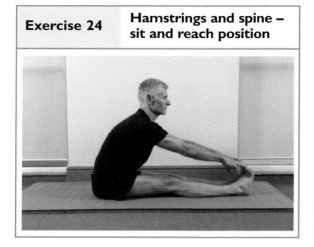

Exercise 25	Hamstrings – standing

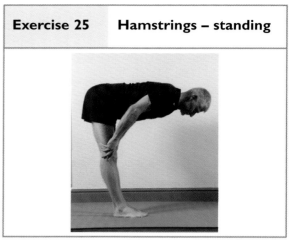

Starting position and instructions

Sit on the floor with your legs straight out in front of you. Reach forwards to touch your toes, curling evenly through the whole of your spine. This exercise stretches the hamstrings and the spine. If an individual is hyperflexible in the thoracic spine, this area will take an excessive stretch. Spinal alignment must be maintained throughout the exercise.

Variations

Start the exercise in the same position with a straight spine, press the chest forwards and retract the shoulders. Move only from the hips using a hinge action. Alternatively, start the exercise with your legs bent and reach forwards as far as you can. Hold this position as you try to straighten first one and then the other leg.

Points to note

The first modification reduces the forwards distance you reach, but increases the stretch on the hamstrings. The second modification reduces the momentum caused by moving the heavy trunk and focuses the stretch more precisely on the hamstrings.

Starting position and instructions

Stand with your feet hip width apart and your knees slightly bent. Bend forwards, keeping your spine as straight as possible so that you move from the hip rather than through the spine. Bend your knee so that you can press your chest against your thighs. Reach around your calves and grip your shins or ankles then, keeping your chest on your knees, try to straighten your legs. Stop at the point where your chest begins to lift from your thighs and hold the position for 20–30 seconds.

Variations

You can practise the same movement sitting on a mat or in a chair. In each case, the movement begins with the chest on the thighs and the aim is to straighten the legs up to the point where the chest begins to lift from the thighs. Hold this position for 20–30 seconds.

Points to note

The standing position is not suitable if you have a history of low-back pain, as it places significant leverage forces on the lumbar region. Choose one of the sitting positions instead. If you find the leg straightening action too intense, hold just one straight first and then the other.

Exercise 26	Flat back hamstring stretch

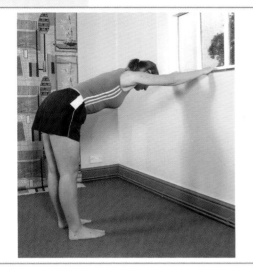

Exercise 27	Hamstrings – sitting

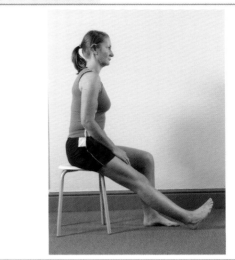

Starting position and instructions

Stand in front of a waist-high object such as a low cupboard or piece of gym equipment with your feet hip width apart and your legs straight. Keeping your trunk very straight, bend forwards at the hips and reach your arms out to rest on the ledge in front of you. Make sure that your hips, shoulders, elbows and hands form a straight line.

Variations

Instead of supporting yourself on a ledge, you can place your hands on your knees or thighs and support your bodyweight through your locked arms.

Points to note

The aim of this movement is to place a stretch on the hamstrings by tilting the pelvis forwards and keeping the spine straight or even slightly hollow (lumbar lordosis maintained). To facilitate this, pull your abdomen in and slightly brace your shoulders while pressing your chest outwards (thoracic extension).

Starting position and instructions

Sit on a bench or stool that allows you to reach the floor with your right leg straight and your left leg bent. Tilt your pelvis forwards and, keeping your spine straight, reach forwards towards your knees. Support your body-weight through your arms throughout the exercise.

Variations

Pulling the foot and toes up towards you and flexing the neck and spine will increase the emphasis on the neural tissues and sciatic nerve.

Points to note

Those who have had back pain may have tightness in the neural tissues or sciatic nerve, which may cause pins and needles during this movement.

Exercise 28	Hamstrings – using a stool

Exercise 29	Hamstrings – using a bench

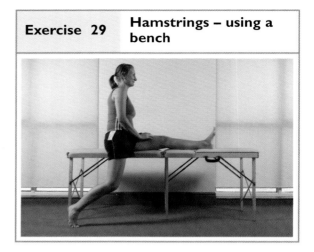

Starting position and instructions

Stand in front of a waist-high stool and place your right foot on it. Keeping your right leg straight, lean forwards, moving from the hip while maintaining correct spinal alignment.

Variations

Hold on to an object or place your hand on a wall to increase the stability of the movement.

Points to note

Pulling your toes towards you and flexing your head and trunk will increase the stretch on the neural tissues and take the stretch away from the hamstring muscles.

Starting position and instructions

Sit with your right leg straight along a bench, and your left leg flexed at the knee and pressed back into extension of the hip. Lean forwards, attempting to reach the foot of your right leg.

Variations

Releasing the full knee extension will increase the emphasis on the upper portion of the hamstrings.

Points to note

The pelvis should not tilt when extending the hip; no more than 15 degrees extension is required.

Exercise 30   Rectus femoris – lying

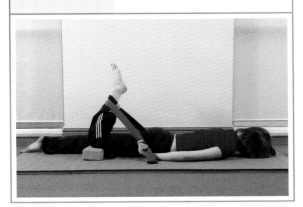

Starting position and instructions

Lie on the floor on your front and bend your right knee. Loop a towel or yoga belt around your right ankle and pull your knee into flexion, drawing your heel towards your buttock.

Variations

Place your knee on a block, forcing the hip into extension. This emphasises the upper portion of the muscle.

Points to note

The upper and lower portion of the muscle must be stretched equally.

Exercise 31   ITB – upper portion

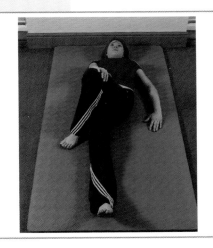

Starting position and instructions

Lie on your back on a mat. Keeping your right foot on the floor, bend your right leg to 90 degrees at the knee and hook your left calf over the top of it. Grip the upper rim of your pelvis with your right hand and, holding your pelvis down on the mat, use your left leg to press your right hip into adduction. Hold the stretched position for 30–60 seconds and then repeat the movement on the other side of the body.

Variations

Altering the amount of hip and knee flexion will vary the effect of the stretch.

Points to note

The ITB (ilio-tibial band) may be tight when the tensor fascia lata muscle that inserts into it is overworked. This can cause pain along the outside of the hip and thigh which this stretch can help to ease. The pain-relieving aspect of this movement can be enhanced by pressing any painful spots (trigger points) along the outer edge of the hip while performing the stretch. Hold the pressure until the pain begins to subside.

| Exercise 32 | ITB – whole length | Exercise 33 | Deep calf and Achilles |

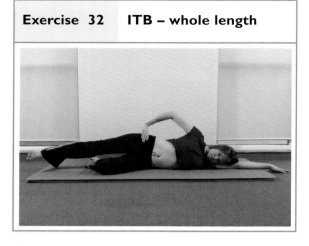

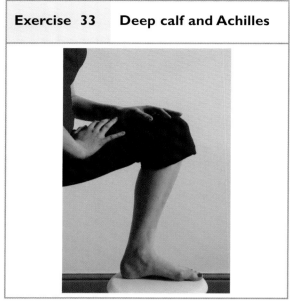

Starting position and instructions

Lie on your left side with your left leg slightly bent for support. Lift your right leg upwards and sideways (abduction) and press the left side of your body firmly into the mat. Keeping the side of your body in contact with the mat, allow the upper leg to lower down onto the mat (adduction).

Variations

Slightly flexing or extending the upper hip (moving it forwards or backwards, respectively) will alter the effect of this movement.

Points to note

The aim of this exercise is to adduct the top hip without allowing the pelvis to tilt sideways. This is achieved by flattening the side of the trunk against the mat and maintaining this position as the stretch is performed. If the pelvis is allowed to move, even slightly, the stretch will be ineffective. If your ITB is flexible, you may not notice this stretch achieving anything. Only when the ITB is tight do you feel the stretch over the outside of the hip. This exercise can also be performed with a partner holding your pelvis level.

Starting position and instructions

Place a low stool or chair against a wall. Put your right foot in the centre of the chair and your left foot on the floor and slightly to the side of the chair and take up a lunge position. Keeping your foot flat, and your heel in contact with the chair seat, press your knee forwards over your toes.

Variations

Altering the angle of the foot away from the perpendicular will change the emphasis on the deep calf and Achilles.

Points to note

The heel must remain on the chair seat throughout the movement. Raising the heel takes the emphasis away from the deep calf and Achilles and throws it onto the foot itself. By bending the knee, the emphasis is taken away from the long superficial calf muscle (gastrocnemius) and placed on the shorter deep calf muscles (soleus and tibialis posterior).

Exercise 34	Side flexion over roll

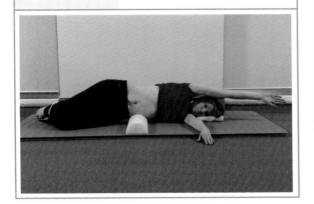

Exercise 35	Whole back extension over gym ball

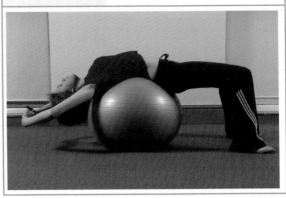

Starting position and instructions

Roll up a bath towel to form a 15–20 cm thick roll. Lie on your side on a mat and place the roll under the side of your trunk, between the rim of your pelvis and your lower ribs. Allow your pelvis and hips to sink down into the mat and reach your upper arm over your head to try to touch the mat. Hold the stretch for 20–30 seconds, breathing normally.

Variations

Crossing your legs and bringing your top leg forwards will allow your pelvis to tip further sideways, increasing the intensity of the stretch.

Points to note

This stretch targets the side flexors of the trunk (obliques and quadratus lumborum) and the latissimus dorsi. To isolate the trunk, keep your arm at your side and do not reach overhead.

Starting position and instructions

Sit on a gym ball with your knees and hips bent to 90 degrees. Your feet should be wider than shoulder width apart and flat on the floor. Walk your feet forwards so that the gym ball rolls under your back and stop when it lies between your shoulder blades. Straighten your arms and reach over your head and back towards the floor, allowing your hips to drop down towards the floor at the same time.

Variations

By adjusting the position of the gym ball, you can determine which area of your spine receives the greatest stretch.

Points to note

This is an extreme stretch, but is quite comfortable to hold as the whole of the spine is supported. If you find the stretch too difficult, deflate the gym ball slightly so that it is flatter and more squashy. The flatter contour of the ball will reduce the intensity of the stretch.

Exercise 36	Thoracic spine over roll	Exercise 37	Toe flexion and extension

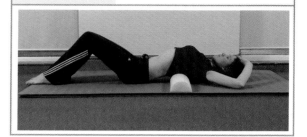

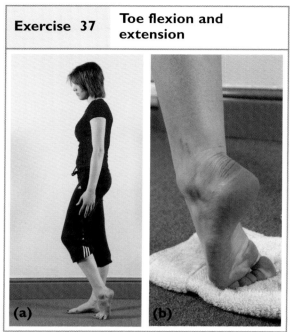

(a)   **(b)**

Starting position and instructions

Lie flat on the floor with your knees bent and feet flat. Have your training partner place a rolled towel beneath your thoracic spine so that the towel runs perpendicular to your spine. Straighten your arms and grip your hands together loosely. Breathe in and raise your arms overhead, trying to touch the mat behind you. As you do so, allow your thoracic spine to be stretched over the towel. Do not lift your spine off the mat.

Variations

Altering the position of the towel will change the focus of the movement. Shuffling up and down will enable you to place the towel at the exact point of stiffness in the thoracic spine. If you find that the towel is uncomfortable, use two small towels and place them end-to-end so that there is a 2 cm gap between them. Place this gap beneath the spinous processes of your back.

Points to note

The exercise can be performed with the legs straight to lengthen the spine along its entire span. However, with the legs straight it is easy to arch the lower back, which in turn takes some of the stretch away from the thoracic spine. If the legs are kept straight, ensure that the hollow beneath the lower back (lumbar lordosis) does not increase.

Starting position and instructions

Stand with your feet bare and your hands against a wall. Point your foot (plantarflex) and press the ball of your foot into a mat (see (a) above), forcing your toes to bend upwards (extend). Hold the position for 10 seconds and then release. Pause, and then press the backs of your toes into the mat (see (b) above), encouraging your toes to bend downwards (flex).

Variations

If you find this stretch uncomfortable, press your toes onto a cushion or folded towel placed on the mat.

Points to note

Encourage this movement, but do not force it. Some individuals may have arthritic changes in their big toe joint (hallux rigidus), which will restrict the free movement of the joint and will require specialist physiotherapy.

Exercise 38   Plantarfascia

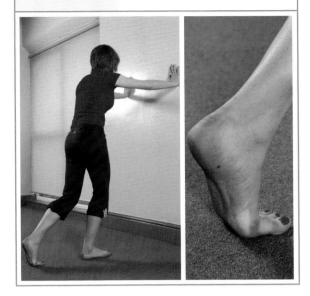

Exercise 39   Peronei muscles

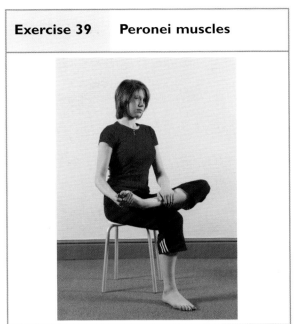

Starting position and instructions

With your feet bare, stand in a supported lunge position with your hands against a wall. Gently press the ball of your foot into a mat, pressing your knee downwards and forwards to encourage plantarflexion of your ankle.

Variations

You can alter the degree of either the knee or toe flexion (or both) to vary this stretch.

Points to note

The plantarfascia in the sole of the foot is tightened by a combination of toe flexion and ankle plantarflexion to wind the fascia around the ball of the foot as the arch of the foot is raised. Both actions combined are required, and either one performed on its own is less effective.

Starting position and instructions

Sit on a bench with your legs crossed, the ankle of your right leg over the knee of the left. Place your right hand on your right shin (medial malleolus) to stabilise the leg, and hook the fingers of your left hand around the outside of your right foot. Draw your foot inwards (inversion) and downwards (plantarflexion) with your left hand as you push against your right ankle with your right hand. Hold this position for 10–20 seconds and then reverse the exercise to stretch the left leg.

Variations

Altering the relative amounts of plantarflexion and inversion of the foot will change the emphasis of the stretch.

Points to note

To take the strain off your fingers, use your forearm and hand to pull your foot inwards, rather than simply the fingers.

Exercise 40	Lower back extension – lying

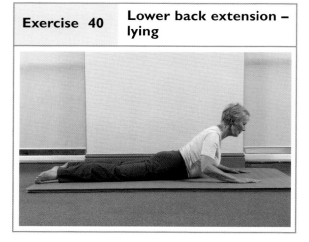

Exercise 41	Thoracic spine rotation – lying

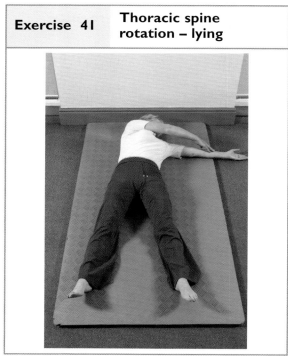

Starting position and instructions

Lie on the floor on your front and place your hands on the floor in the 'press-up' position. Push with your arms to arch your spine, keeping your hips firmly on the floor. Pause in the upper position and then lower. This movement stretches the rectus abdominis muscle and corrects any pressure imbalance in the lower back discs caused by prolonged sitting or lifting.

Variations

Pushing from your forearms until your elbows are locked at 90 degrees will limit the range of motion; pulling your arms towards your shoulders will increase the range of motion.

Points to note

This movement should be encouraged rather than forced, and repeated rhythmically to gain a pumping action on the discs of your lower spine. You should feel the stretch, but not pain, in the lower back. If you experience pain, stop immediately.

Starting position and instructions

Lie on the floor with your legs comfortably apart, and your arms out in a 'T' position. Stretch your right arm across your body aiming to touch your left hand and rotate your trunk to the left at the same time. This movement stretches the thoracic spine and the oblique abdominals and latissimus dorsi muscles of the upper side of the body.

Variations

Increasing the amount of abduction of your legs will increase the stability of the movement.

Points to note

Keeping your hips still will increase the emphasis of the stretch on your thoracic spine.

Exercise 42	Full spine rotation – standing

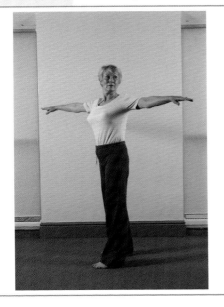

Exercise 43	Spinal rotation – using a stick

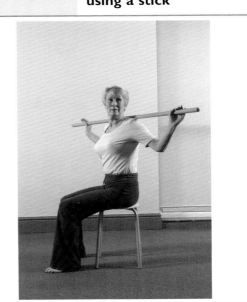

Starting position and instructions

Stand with your feet astride and arms out in a 'T' position. Rotate to the right, leading with your right arm, and then reverse the movement. This exercise stretches the oblique abdominals.

Variations

Lowering your arms and leading just with the shoulders reduces the overload.

Points to note

The leverage and momentum from your arms make it essential that the movement is performed in a slow and controlled fashion.

Starting position and instructions

Sit astride a bench with a stick across your shoulders. Grip the ends of the stick and twist your trunk to the right, pressing your right elbow backwards and your left elbow forwards. This movement stretches the oblique abdominals.

Variations

Reaching your hands above your head before beginning the stretch will pull harder on the thoracolumbar fascia.

Points to note

This exercise must be performed slowly, with a hold at the end to avoid building up potentially damaging momentum. If your shoulder flexibility does not permit you to place the stick across your shoulders, hold it on the front of the chest at the level of the upper part of your breastbone.

Exercise 44	Spinal rotation – lying: (a) normal (b) extreme movement range

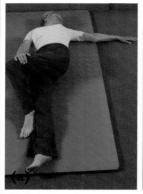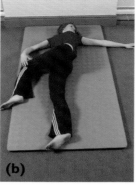

Starting position and instructions

Lie on the floor with your right arm out at 90 degrees. Flex your right knee and rotate your trunk towards the left leg, bringing your right knee towards the floor. Place overpressure on the stretch by pressing your knee to the floor using your left arm. The main emphasis of this stretch is on the oblique abdominals, but it also stretches the latissimus dorsi and anterior deltoid of the horizontal arm.

Variations

If you find the stretch too difficult place a cushion on the floor and take your knee down on to the cushion. Alternatively, altering the degree of flexion at your hip and knee will alter the stress of the stretch.

Points to note

Because this action involves leverage, it should be performed in a slow and controlled manner. As the rotation occurs, the lower hip will tuck under the body. This is desirable, as it becomes the pivot point around which the body moves.

Exercise 45	Spinal rotation – two legs: (a) normal (b) extreme movement range

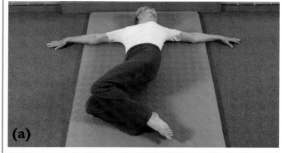
(a)

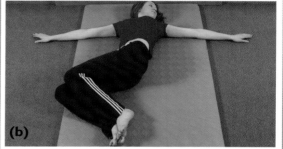
(b)

Starting position and instructions

Lie on the floor with your knees and hips flexed. Take your knees to the right side of your body and your arms to the left, maintaining the stretch. The main emphasis of this stretch is on the oblique abdominals, but it also stretches the latissimus dorsi and anterior deltoid of the upper arm.

Variations

Place a small cushion on the floor and lower your knees on to the cushion to reduce the range of motion.

Points to note

Due to the weight of your legs, they should be lowered slowly; dropping your legs is potentially dangerous to your spine.

Exercise 46	Spinal rotation – sitting (assisted)

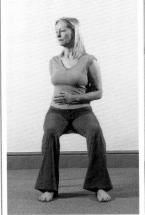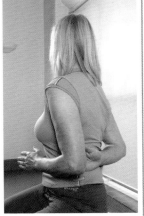

Starting position and instructions

Sit on a low bench, place your right arm behind the small of your back and grip the elbow of your left arm with your right hand. Twist to the right, leading the movement with the left hand. This exercise stretches the oblique abdominals.

Variations

If you are unable to grip your elbow, a looped towel may be used around the elbow instead.

Points to note

It is usual to have some degree of asymmetry, so rotation to the right and left sides may not be equal.

Exercise 47	Lateral flexion – standing

Right **Wrong**

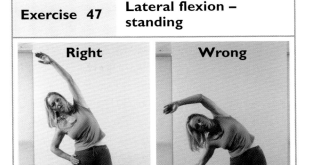

Starting position and instructions

Stand with your feet astride. Laterally flex your spine, placing your left arm on your waist or thigh to support your body-weight. Take your right arm above your head to increase the stretch. This movement stretches the latissimus dorsi and external oblique on the right side of the body.

Variations

Place both arms on the waist to reduce the overload. Stretching both hands overhead increases the overload on the spine, and changes the emphasis of the exercise from stretch to strength.

Points to note

Asymmetry of the lateral flexion of the spine is common, so movements may not be equal on both sides.

Exercise 48	Lateral flexion – using a stick

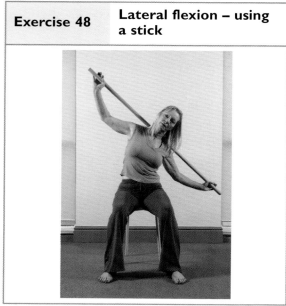

Exercise 49	Lateral flexion – with overpressure

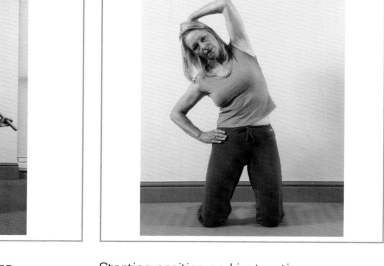

Starting position and instructions

Sit astride a bench with a stick across your shoulders. Grip the ends of the stick and laterally flex to the right, moving the stick upwards towards the ceiling. This movement stretches the external oblique and quadratus lumborum on the left side of the body.

Variations

A towel can be used instead of the stick if your shoulder is not flexible enough to allow the stick to be placed behind your neck. Alternatively, hold the stick on your chest at the level of the upper part of your breastbone.

Points to note

Pure lateral flexion should be used rather than combining it with flexion or rotation. In addition, the pivot point of the movement should be at the level of the breastbone (sternum) rather than at the waist. Pivoting around the breastbone keeps the body upright, while pivoting around the waist causes the body to lean sideways.

Starting position and instructions

Kneel on the floor and reach above your head with your right arm to lead a lateral flexion movement. Your left arm acts as a pivot by pressing the side of your ribcage. This exercise stretches the external oblique and the quadratus lumborum on the right side of the body.

Variations

Instead of taking your arm above your head, place both arms on your hips to reduce the overload on your spine.

Points to note

Asymmetry in this area is common so movements may not be equal on both sides.

Exercise 50	Trunk lateral shift

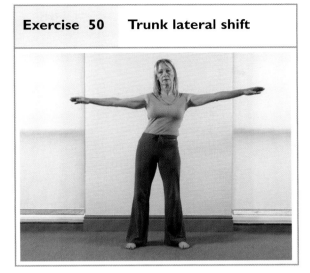

Exercise 51	Trunk lateral shift – against a wall

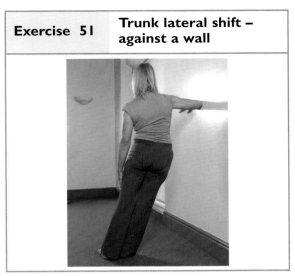

Starting position and instructions

Stand with your arms out in a 'T' position. Lunge to the side with your right hand to shift the trunk. This exercise stretches the external oblique and quadratus lumborum on the left side of the body.

Variations

Performing the exercise with your back against a wall will ensure maximum alignment; performing in front of a mirror will often make the movement easier to control.

Points to note

The movement should come from your hips, with your shoulders remaining fairly static.

Starting position and instructions

Stand right side on to a wall with your right arm abducted to 90 degrees, your elbow bent and your forearm supported on the wall. Keep your shoulders still and press the right side of your pelvis and hips towards the wall.

Variations

If your posture type means that your spine leans more to one side than the other, perform the exercise only on that side. This is because the side flexor muscles on the side you lean towards will be shorter, and therefore require more stretching. For example, if your spine leans to the right, your right side flexor muscles will be tighter than those on the left. Pressing the pelvis to the right is actually equivalent to leaning over to the left (when the shoulders move to the left, the pelvis moves to the right), which stretches the right side of the body.

Points to note

There is very little movement in this exercise, so the action is one of a subtle press or squeeze rather than a noticeable muscle stretch.

Exercise 52	Skull rock

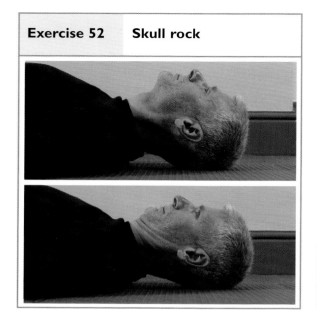

Exercise 53	Cervical spine flexion – with overpressure

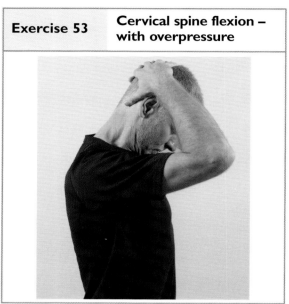

Starting position and instructions

Lie on your back on a mat. Relax your shoulders and keep the back of your head on the mat throughout the movement. Gently draw your chin in, as though trying to press your chin into the top of your breastbone.

Variations

This exercise can also be performed while standing, with your head and shoulders resting against a wall. Also, to increase the effect of the stretch you can assist the movement by placing overpressure on your chin with your hands. This movement emphasises the stretch on the upper part of the cervical spine.

Points to note

As you perform this action, the back of the skull should move in a line up and down the mat by about 10 cm. If you find that your head does not rest on the mat easily, place one or two thin books underneath your head until the resting position suits your posture.

Starting position and instructions

Sit on a gym bench, interlace your fingers and place your hands behind your head. Bend your neck to look downwards towards your chest, then place overpressure on this movement by pulling gently on the back of your head with your hands. Maintain the stretched position for 10 seconds and then repeat. Perform three repetitions only.

Variations

You can also stretch the upper part of the thoracic spine by allowing the shoulders to round slightly. To restrict the movement to the upper cervical spine, try to draw the chin into the lower part of the throat instead of looking down at the chest.

Points to note

As the neck is a delicate structure, the overpressure used in this stretch must be small and controlled. Use very light pressure from the hands to guide the neck, rather than forcing the movement. Do not perform high repetitions of this movement; three is the maximum required.

Exercise 54	Cervical rotation – with overpressure

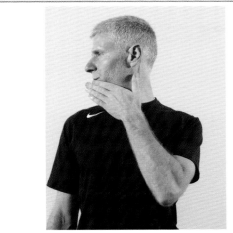

Exercise 55	Jaw joint

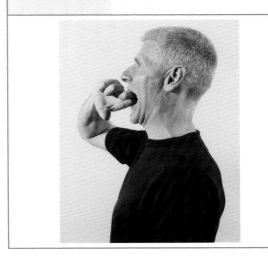

Starting position and instructions

Sit on a gym bench with your spine correctly aligned. Turn your head to the right and assist the movement by gently pressing onto the angle of your jaw with your left hand. Aim to bring your chin over the point of your shoulder.

Variations

The rotation movement can also be combined with either flexion (look down towards the floor) or extension (look up at the ceiling).

Points to note

As you turn your head, be careful not to turn your trunk as well by twisting the shoulders, as this will release some of the stretch. The neck should move relative to the shoulders, not with them.

Starting position and instructions

Sit in front of a mirror. Open your mouth and place one bent finger between your teeth. Maintain this stretch for 10–20 seconds and then remove the finger and close your mouth. Repeat the stretch, this time using two fingers and, eventually (after many weeks), using three.

Variations

If your jaw is so tight that you are unable to even get one finger between your teeth, use a thinner object such as a toothbrush handle at first.

Points to note

The jaw joint (tempero mandibular joint or TMJ) is controlled by the powerful biting muscles. In individuals who have a tendency to grind their teeth at night, these muscles become short and tight. To stretch them effectively may take weeks, gradually increasing the movement by a few millimetres each day. As the stretch is placed on the joint, try to relax the jaw and allow the stretch to take effect. Avoid the temptation to actually 'bite' the finger and tense the jaw muscles.

Exercise 56	Rhomboids and thoracic spine

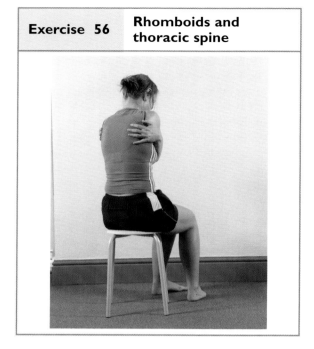

Exercise 57	Anterior chest and shoulders

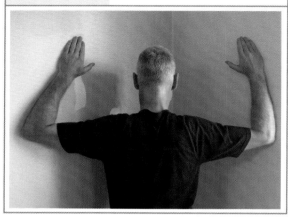

Starting position and instructions

Stand in front of a doorway or in the corner of a room with your shoulders and elbows flexed to 90 degrees. Lean forwards, pressing your chest through the doorway and forcing your arms back into extension.

Variations

Increasing and reducing the height of the arms will vary the focus of the stretch.

Points to note

Because the full body-weight is being supported, heavy individuals and those with poor shoulder flexibility should take up a lunge position, moving some of the body-weight on to the front foot.

Starting position and instructions

Sitting on a bench, cross your arms across your chest placing your hand on the opposite shoulder, and flex your trunk at the thoracic spine.

Variations

Combine the flexion movement with rotation and/or lateral flexion to change the emphasis on the thoracic spine. If you feel pain between your shoulder blades that is relieved by this movement, the pain is often caused by spasms within the rhomboid muscles. Pain relief can be enhanced by having someone gently press their thumbs into the muscles between the spine and the inner (medial) edge of the scapula while in the stretched position.

Points to note

This exercise should be used with caution, as this area of the spine is quite often too flexible (hyperflexible).

Exercise 58	Pectoralis – minor muscle

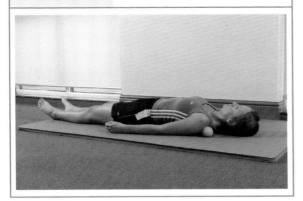

Starting position and instructions

Lie on your back on a mat. Tuck your right hand beneath the outside of your right hip and place a small ball such as a squash ball between the back of your right shoulder and the mat. The squash ball should be level with the ball of the joint rather than your shoulder blade. Firmly press your shoulder backwards, trying to compress the squash ball. Hold the stretched position for 20–30 seconds and then release.

Variations

Pressing on to a squash ball is an active stretch and requires the strength of your shoulder retractor muscles to be greater than the tightness of your shoulder protractor muscles. However, if your shoulder is very tight, it may be better to perform the exercise passively by asking your training partner to press your shoulder down using the flat of their hand.

Points to note

As you perform the action try not to rotate the trunk and ribcage to the side as this will release the stretching force. Instead, keep the ribcage relatively fixed, as the shoulder is stretched.

Exercise 59	Upper trapezius

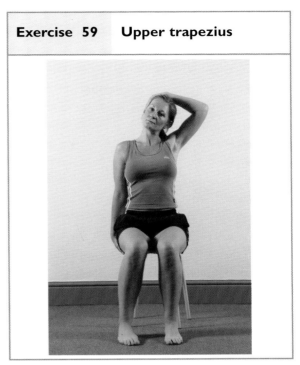

Starting position and instructions

Sit on a bench and grip the bench top with your right hand. Laterally flex your neck to the left allowing your right shoulder to elevate. Fix your neck in position with your left hand, and actively depress your right shoulder to overload the stretch.

Variations

Flex and extend your head to change the emphasis of the stretch.

Points to note

The power from the stretch must be from pulling the shoulder downwards rather than pulling on the neck, since the neck is the more delicate structure.

Exercise 60	Upper trapezius – with band

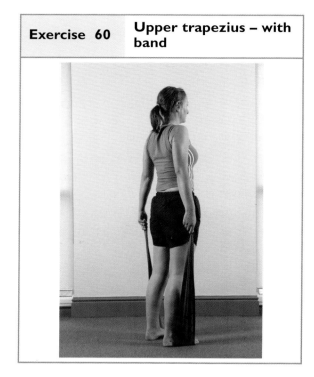

Exercise 61	Shoulder adductors and extensors

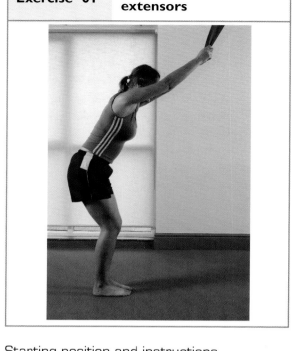

Starting position and instructions

Stand of the floor holding a band in both hands. Place the band beneath your feet and stand upright. Shrug your shoulders against the resistance of the band, then let the band draw your shoulders down and slightly backwards.

Variations

A heavier resistance band can be used for a greater stretch.

Points to note

The emphasis should be on the stretch, so shrug the shoulders for two counts and allow four counts for the band to stretch the shoulders downwards. Make sure that you maintain your spinal alignment throughout this movement; do not allow the band to pull you down into flexion.

Starting position and instructions

Grip a high point and straighten your arms. Keeping your hands fixed, bend your knees and lower your body down and back, feeling the stretch beneath your arms. This movement stretches the latissimus dorsi and the triceps muscles.

Variations

Altering the position of the hands will change the exact point of the stretch.

Points to note

Gripping a higher point will increase the range of motion, but reduce the bodyweight placed on the stretch. Gripping a lower point will encourage you to lean back and take more weight through your shoulders.

Exercise 62	Shoulder rotation – lying

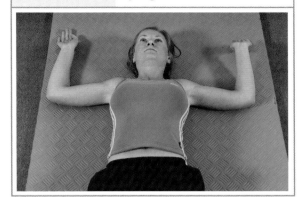

Exercise 63	Shoulder rotation – weight overload

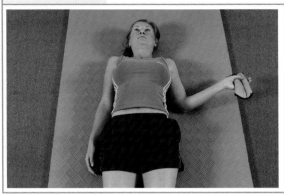

Starting position and instructions

Lie on the floor with your arms abducted and elbows flexed to 90 degrees. Allow your forearms to fall back into the horizontal position, rotating the shoulders. This position stretches the shoulder rotators.

Variations

Alter the angle of abduction at the shoulder to vary the exact site of the stretch.

Points to note

With the use of weights, this exercise is ideal for contract–relax techniques.

Starting position and instructions

Lie on the floor and grip a weight bag in your right hand. Place your upper arm close to your body and flex your elbow to 90 degrees. Allow the weight of the bag to force your shoulder into external rotation. This position stretches the shoulder rotators.

Variations

Increasing and reducing the weight will change the intensity of the stretch.

Points to note

Since a weight is used, this exercise is ideal for contract–relax techniques. Try to ensure that the shoulder does not move forwards as the stretch is placed on the shoulder. Keep the back of the shoulder in contact with the mat throughout the movement.

Exercise 64	Forearm pronation and wrist flexion

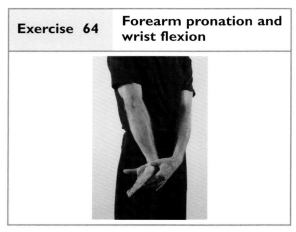

Starting position and instructions

Stand with your arms by your sides. Pronate your right forearm and flex your right wrist. Grip your right wrist with your left hand and press your right wrist into further flexion.

Variations

This exercise can be combined with radial or ulnar deviation to maximally stress your extensor carpi radialis longus muscle.

Points to note

For cases of tennis elbow, combining the wrist flexion and ulnar deviation will maximally stress your extensor carpi radialis longus muscle.

Exercise 65	Forearm pronation and supination – using a stick

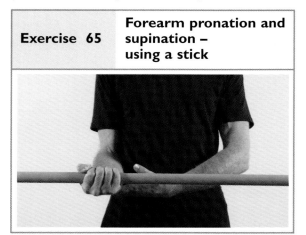

Starting position and instructions

Flex your right elbow and turn your forearm so that your palm faces upwards. Gripping a stick in your right hand, support your forearm in your cupped left hand. Pronate and supinate your right forearm, using the weight of the stick as overpressure.

Variations

Using a lighter or heavier stick will change the intensity of the stretch.

Points to note

Holding the stretch at the end of the range of motion will increase the overload.

Exercise 66	Wrist extensors – on a table

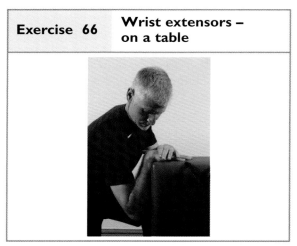

Starting position and instructions

Place your right hand at the edge of a low table and place your left hand on top of your right so that your thumb is level with your wrist crease. Press the right forearm down into the vertical position, pressing your right wrist into extension. Use the weight from your left hand to keep the heel of your right hand on the table.

Variations

Altering the height of the table will vary the range of motion of the wrist.

Points to note

Where a single intercarpel joint is stiff, the movement can be localised by pressing the thumb of the left hand into the wrist crease of the right hand.

Exercise 67	**Wrist extensors – with self overpressure**

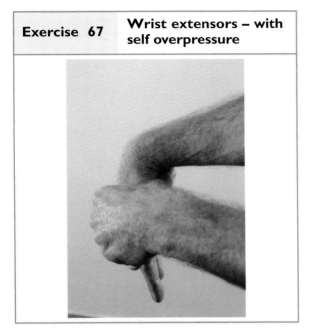

Starting position and instructions

Straighten your right arm and flex your right wrist. Grip your right hand with your left, placing your left thumb into the crease of your right wrist. Using your left thumb as a pivot, pull your right wrist into full flexion.

Variations

Altering the position of the thumb will localise the stretch.

Points to note

Because of the leverage involved, the stretch must be slow and controlled.

Exercise 68	**Wrist extensors – against a wall**

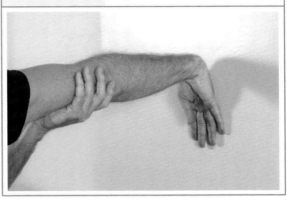

Starting position and instructions

Stand facing a wall, place the back of your right hand flat on the wall with your fingers vertical and straighten your arm. Use your left hand to lock your right elbow and maintain the locked position throughout the movement. Lean forwards towards the wall, pressing your wrist into further flexion.

Variations

Placing your hand higher up the wall will increase the range of motion.

Points to note

Where an ache is felt close to the elbow, the muscle is being stretched, but where the sensation is over the wrist, the wrist extensor tendons and tissue are being stretched.

127

Exercise 69	Wrist flexors

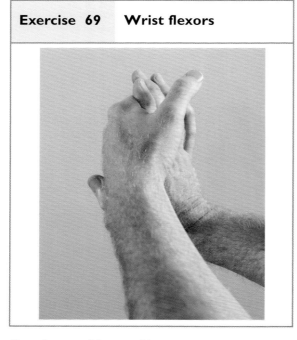

Starting position and instructions

Straighten your right arm and, with your left hand, take hold of the palm of your right hand below the knuckles and pull your right hand back in to extension. Hold the stretch for 10 seconds and then repeat.

Variations

Placing the thumb of the left hand in the crease at the back of the right hand will localise the stretch to the area of the wrist.

Points to note

There are seven small carpal bones within the wrist; this exercise will stretch all of the wrist, but will not isolate the stretch to a single bone. If a single joint is stiff, manual therapy from a physiotherapist will be required before the stretch is placed on.

Exercise 70	Wrist abduction and adduction

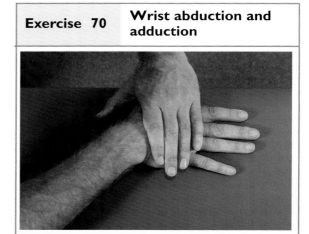

Starting position and instructions

Place your right forearm on a low table with your hand flat and fingers spread. Place your left hand over your right to prevent your hand from sliding on the tabletop. Glide your forearm from side to side, encouraging abduction and adduction at the wrist.

Variations

Both abduction and adduction can be combined with a slight amount of flexion or extension to vary the stretch.

Points to note

There is always more adduction (movement towards the little finger) than abduction (movement towards the thumb) available at the wrist.

Exercise 71   Finger flexors

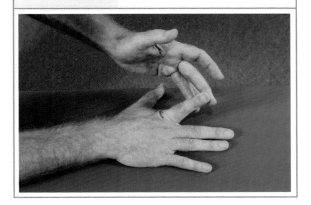

Starting position and instructions

Grip one finger of your right hand, placing your left thumb on the first metacarpophalangeal joint. Place the forefinger of your left hand underneath the right finger. Pull the finger back into extension. Repeat on all fingers.

Variations

Combining extension with abduction and adduction will vary the site of the stretch.

Points to note

Because of the leverage involved, the stretch must be slow and controlled.

Exercise 72   Finger flexors and palm of the hand

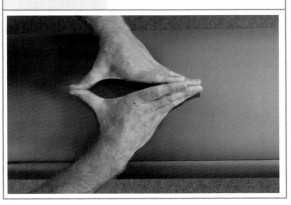

Starting position and instructions

Place the tips of your fingers and thumbs together. Press your hands closer together to force your fingers and thumbs into extension. Hold the stretch for 10 seconds and then repeat.

Variations

Because the tissues being stretched are superficial, heat will increase the range of motion. The exercise can therefore be performed with the hands submerged in warm water.

Points to note

Individuals who have extremely lax finger joints may find that their distal interphalangeal joint hyperextends. If this is the case, they should start with the fingers flexed first and then stretch to the mid-position only.

Exercise 73	Finger adductors

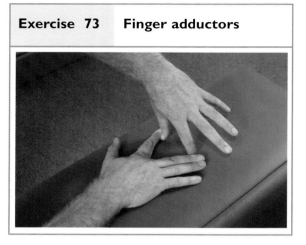

Starting position and instructions

Place your right hand on a flat surface and place two fingers of your left hand between two of the right. Force the right-hand fingers apart.

Variations

A small golf ball can be used between your fingers instead of your other hand. Pressing the golf ball closer to the web of your hand increases the range of motion obtained with the stretch.

Points to note

Because of the leverage involved, the stretch must be slow and controlled. In individuals where the distal interphalangeal joints are hyper-mobile, the stretch can be placed closer to the finger web.

ADVANCED STRETCHES

Exercise 74	**Hip flexors and extensors – modified lunge**

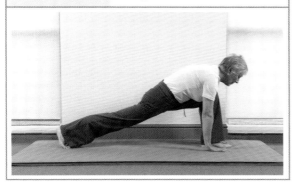

Exercise 75	**Hip flexors and extensors – extended range**

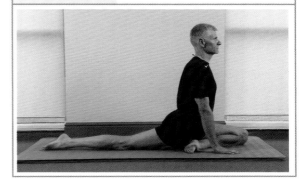

Starting position and instructions

Start with your feet shoulder width apart. Step forwards with your right leg and lower your body towards the ground, supporting your weight with your hands. Keep your right foot flat and your knee and foot in line.

Variations

Placing the hands inside the knee will increase the available range of motion.

Points to note

Because full body-weight is being used, the exercise must be performed slowly.

Starting position and instructions

Start with your feet shoulder width apart. Step forwards with your right leg and lower your body towards the ground, supporting your weight with your hands. Turn your right knee outwards and your right foot inwards to bring the right thigh down onto the ground, with the right heel on the inside of your groin. At the same time, slide your left leg backwards to bring it down onto the mat.

Variations

Bending your left knee will increase the stretch on the rectus femoris of your left leg. Instead of turning your right knee out and bringing your heel to the inside of the groin, you can simply sit on the heel of your right leg. This reduces the stretch on the gluteal muscles of the right leg, but also takes away any rotation strain on the knee.

Points to note

This is an extreme stretch and as such should only be practised after the basic stretch for the hip flexors and extensors (*see* exercise 73) has been mastered. The exercise should be performed slowly, keeping control of the body-weight at all times by lowering the body with the hands.

Exercise 76	Hip adductors – standing

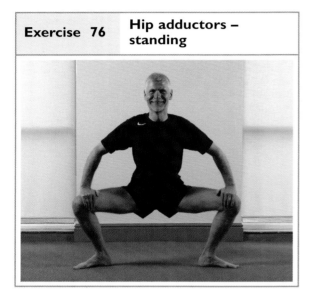

Starting position and instructions

Stand with your feet astride and your toes pointing out. Squat down until your thighs are at 90 degrees degrees, placing your hands on your knees. Press with your hands to force your knees into further abduction.

Variations

Hold on to your ankle and press your knees apart with your elbows.

Points to note

This movement is quite unstable, so some individuals may find it easier to support their weight on a stool.

Exercise 77	Hip adductors – with trunk lateral flexion

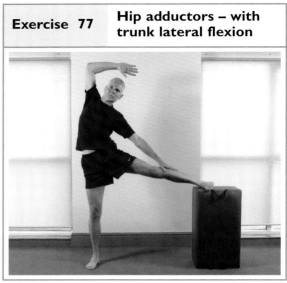

Starting position and instructions

Place your right foot on a waist-high object with your toes pointing forwards and laterally flex your trunk to the right.

Variations

Altering the height of the object will vary the stretch. Taking the left arm overhead will increase the stretch.

Points to note

Because you are standing on one leg, this exercise is unstable; if you need to, hold on to an object throughout the movement. The upper arm must reach towards the foot, not press downwards on the outside of the knee. Because of the stress placed on the knee, this exercise is unsuitable if you have had a knee ligament injury.

Exercise 78	Hip adductors and rotators

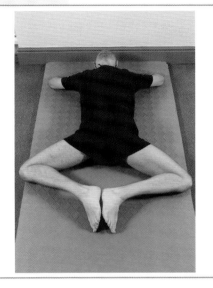

leverage forces are quite high. In children, any movement that forces the hip can be dangerous and if pain occurs in the hip joint rather than in the muscles, the movement must be stopped immediately. In seniors, this movement should not be attempted if you have had a hip joint replacement or hip surgery of any type.

Exercise 79	Gluteals

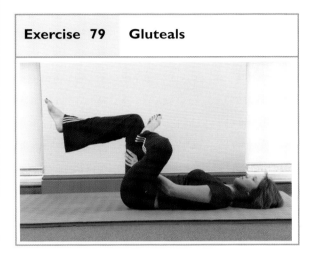

Starting position and instructions

Lie on your front in the 'frog' position: your hips should be flexed, abducted and laterally rotated (turned out). Your knees should be bent to 90 degrees and your feet should be touching. From this position, try to straighten your legs and touch the floor with your toes, without allowing the front of your hips to leave the mat.

Variations

Rather than beginning with your hips on the mat and attempting to touch the mat with your toes, you can begin with your toes on the mat (in which case your hips will lift off the mat) and attempt to lower your hips down. As the hips are heavier than the shins, this action gives greater overpressure.

Points to note

This exercise causes extreme 'turn out' (hip lateral rotation) and so is popular with ballet students. However, it must be used with caution as the

Starting position and instructions

Lie on your back on the floor, flex your right hip and rotate it. Draw your left knee up, pressing your knee on to your right foot. Reach around your left knee and pull your knee towards your shoulder, forcing your right hip into external rotation.

Variations

Altering the angle of hip motion of your left leg will change the emphasis of the stretch.

Points to note

This exercise also places stress on the pelvis, so it is inappropriate after pregnancy. If you are unable to flex your hip high enough to grip around your thigh, loop a towel around your thigh and grip that instead.

Exercise 80	Hamstrings and hip adductors – lying

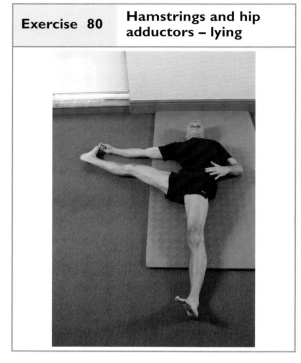

Starting position and instructions

Lie on your back on the floor with both legs straight. Take your right leg into flexion and then out into abduction, aiming to rest it on the floor. Keep both shoulders and hips on the floor.

Variations

Place a small cushion or block under your leg to limit the full movement.

Points to note

The subject must be strong to lower the leg under control, and under no circumstances should the leg be dropped rapidly towards the floor.

Exercise 81	Hamstrings and hip adductors – splits position with stool support

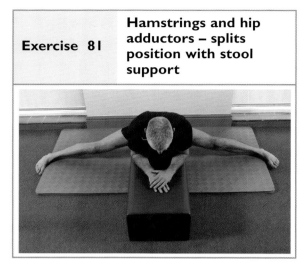

Starting position and instructions

Stand with your feet astride and then slide your feet apart to form a splits position. Flex your trunk at the hip and place your forearms on a stool or 2–3 yoga blocks to support your body-weight.

Variations

Place your feet on a shiny piece of paper (on a carpet surface) or cloth (on a wooden floor) to allow your feet to slide more easily. If you are very flexible, you may be able to dispense with the stool and place your forearms flat on the floor. However, if you do this make sure that you maintain your spinal alignment; do not perform extreme spinal flexion simply to put your arms on the floor. It is better to use a stool and maintain spinal alignment. The effect on hip flexibility is the same in both cases.

Points to note

Your pelvis should remain above your hips throughout the movement and your body-weight must be taken on your forearms to reduce the stress on your knees. This exercise is unsuitable if you have had a knee ligament injury, as it stresses the inner (medial) ligament of the knee.

Exercise 82	Hamstrings and hip adductors – splits position to head

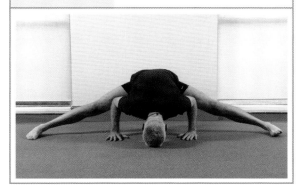

Starting position and instructions

This is a progression to exercise 80 and should only be performed when that exercise can be practised easily. Stand with your feet astride, then slide your feet apart to form a maximal splits position. Take your body-weight back on to your heels and flex your trunk at the hip, bending forwards to take hold of your ankles and then to place your head on the ground.

Variations

Initially, you may find this exercise easier if you sit on a low stool or 3–4 yoga blocks stacked on top of each other.

Points to note

It is essential to take your body-weight backwards on to your heels in this movement. As you place your head on to the ground, at least $\frac{2}{3}$ of your body-weight should be supported by your legs and $\frac{1}{3}$ by your head, purely for balance. This is an extreme movement that is popular with dancers, gymnasts and martial artists. It requires excellent muscle strength and muscle control and should not be attempted by people with poor fitness levels. Even when performed by optimally fit individuals, this stretch places considerable strain on the inner (medial) ligament of the knee. A single repetition only should be performed and held for 10–30 secs maximum.

Exercise 83	Spinal rotation – using leg leverage

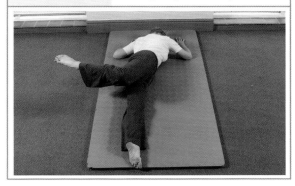

Starting position and instructions

Lie on your front with your head supported by your crossed arms. Take your right leg up and across your body to touch the floor on your left, twisting your trunk and flexing your knee as the movement progresses. This exercise stretches the oblique abdominals.

Variations

Altering the degree of flexion at your knee and the extension of your hip will change the emphasis of the stretch.

Points to note

Due to the weight of your leg, it should be lowered under control rather than forcing your spine into extension and rotation.

| Exercise 84 | Full spine rotation – with overpressure | Exercise 85 | lateral flexion and rotation |

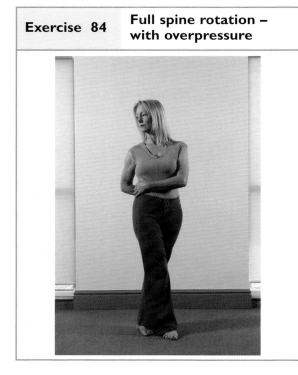

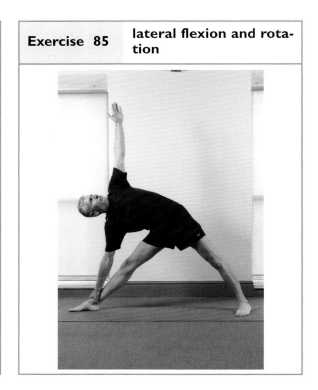

Starting position and instructions

Stand with your feet slightly apart. Cross your right foot over your left to rotate your pelvis and hips to the left. Twist your trunk to the right, bringing your left arm in front of you and your right arm behind you. Grip the inside of your left elbow with your right hand and useyour left arm to pull your right side into further rotation.

Variations

If lack of shoulder flexibility limits your ability to grip your elbow, fold a towel around your left elbow to grip instead.

Points to note

The overpressure that this exercise can generate is quite high. Be careful therefore to keep the action slow and controlled throughout, avoiding the tendency to 'bounce' into the movement.

Starting position and instructions

Stand with your feet astride and turn your right foot out (lateral rotation of the hip). Reach down towards your right shin or ankle with your right arm and point your left arm towards the ceiling to offer counterbalance. This exercise stretches the oblique abdominals and the quadratus lumborum.

Variations

Allow your upper arm to rest on your body to alter the stress.

Points to note

Your body-weight must be taken through your arm on to your shin or ankle throughout the movement to reduce the leverage (stress) on your spine. If you have a history of lower back pain, you should only attempt this exercise under the supervision of a qualified instructor.

Exercise 86   The Triangle

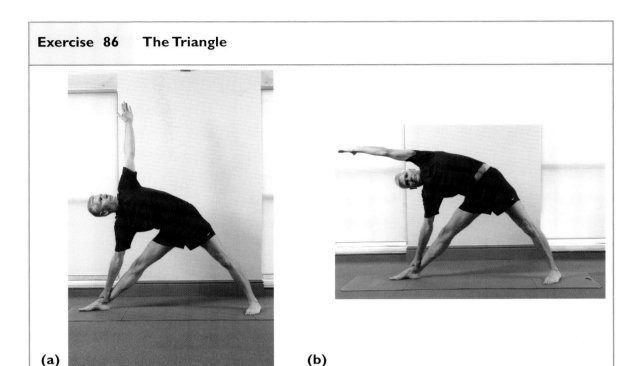

(a)   **(b)**

Starting position and instructions

The triangle is a classic yoga position called *Trikonasana*. Begin with your feet 3–4 times shoulder width apart. Keeping your arms straight, slide your right arm down the outside of your right thigh to the outside of your knee, at the same time reaching your left arm overhead and then to the right. Maintain the position, breathing normally, and press your right hand onto the side of your knee to come back up.

Variations

You can increase the stretch by sliding the right hand further down the leg to the shin or ankle and reaching the left arm up, pointing the fingers to the ceiling. This is a yoga position called the Extended Triangle or *Utthita Trikonasana*.

Points to note

As with exercise 84 it is important that your lower arm takes your body-weight to reduce the strain on the spine. If you release your arm, the trunk muscles alone support the whole of your upper body-weight, changing the movement from a pure stretch to a combination of stretch and strength.

Exercise 87   Lateral flexion and side lunge

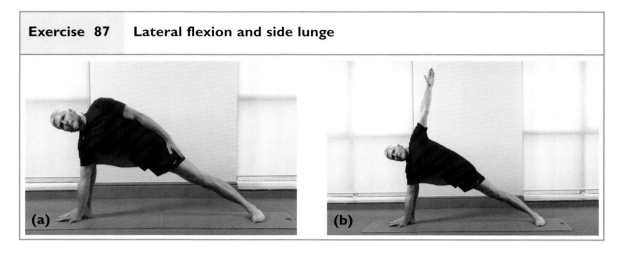

Starting position and instructions

This movement combines lateral flexion of the trunk with a lunge movement (*see* exercise 73) and forms a classic yoga posture called the Side Angle pose or *Parsvakonasana*. Stand with your feet 2–3 times shoulder width apart. Turn your right foot through 90 degrees (lateral rotation of the hip) and your left foot slightly in (medial rotation of the hip). Bend your right knee until your right shin is vertical, keeping your knee directly over your foot. Bend slightly to the right until you are able to rest the right side of your trunk on the top of your right thigh. Support yourself with your right hand on the floor outside your foot. Reach overhead and try to create a straight line from your left leg up the side of your body to your left arm.

Variations

If you are unable to put your right hand flat on the floor, 'tent' your fingers (take the weight on your fingertips) or rest your hand on a yoga block or low stool.

Points to note

Balance is essential in this exercise. If you find yourself wobbling, that means the stretch is un-controlled. This can occur if you are unable to place your hand on the floor as a third point of contact. If this is the case, it is important to use a block or stool for support.

Exercise 88	Back flexion – on gym ball

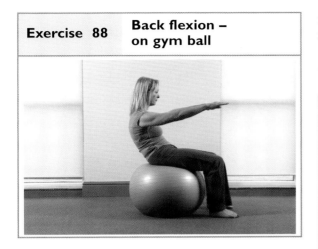

more difficult. If you find that you wobble noticeably during the movement, place a chair or gym bench in front of you and hold onto that as you move.

Exercise 89	Lower back extension – standing

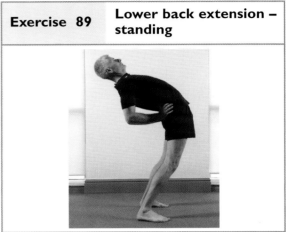

Starting position and instructions

Sit on a gym ball large enough to allow your hips to be slightly above your knees, keeping your knees just wider than shoulder width apart. As you sit, you are on your sitting bones (ischial tuberosities). Tilt your pelvis backwards so that you are sitting more on your tailbone and allow your lower back to bend (flex). Pause in this stretched position, then tilt your pelvis forwards so that you are sitting on your pubic bone, a little like riding a horse.

Variations

You can involve the whole spine in the stretch by bending to look at your umbilicus (belly button) as you tilt your pelvis backwards to sit on your tail. As you tilt your pelvis forwards to sit on your pubic bone, look upwards towards the ceiling and arch (hollow) the whole of your back.

Points to note

Try to avoid 'body sway' when performing the movement, as it makes you less stable on the ball. The aim should be to keep your shoulders over the top of your hips throughout. Placing your hands on your knees will aid your balance; having them out to the sides makes the balance

Starting position and instructions

Stand with your feet hip width apart and your hands at the top of your buttocks. Extend your spine by pressing your hips forwards, pushing with your hands and at the same time looking upwards. Perform the exercise slowly and rhythmically, but do not hold it in the upward position as this is quite stressful on the lower back.

Variations

This action (lumbar extension) can be combined with rotation and/or lateral flexion if the combined movement seems to be stiffer than the pure movement.

Points to note

When the action is stiff and painful, perform it for 3–5 repetitions only. If the pain subsides, the exercise can be continued; if the pain does not subside, rest and then repeat the action; if the pain increases, stop immediately. If you do not press the hips forwards, the extension action becomes a simple 'lean back'. Because of the effect of the gravity line of the body, this places more compression on the lumbar spine than performing the action by moving the hips forwards.

Exercise 90	The Warrior

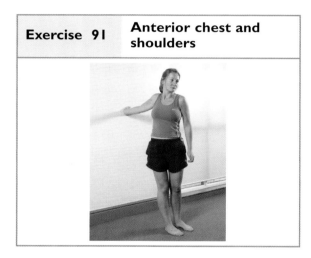

Starting position and instructions

Stand in a stride position with your right foot facing forwards and your left foot turned out by 45–60 degrees (lateral rotation of the hip). Stretch your right arm forwards and your left arm backwards, both along the horizontal. Lunge forwards until your right knee passes over your right foot, lowering your body-weight so that your front thigh is horizontal. Keep your body upright and your arms lengthened.

Variations

Instead of stretching your arms along the horizontal, you can reach your arms overhead, hooking your thumbs together and stretching your fingertips towards the ceiling. Alternatively, you can turn your body and stretch forwards with your left arm and backwards with your right (the Reverse Warrior).

Points to note

This is a classic yoga posture called *Virabhadrasana*. Although it is an excellent exercise, it must be modified if it causes pain. Likely areas of stress are the inside of the knee of the back leg, and lack of flexibility of the ankle of the back leg. In addition, if hip flexibility is poor, the lumbar spine may compensate by hyper-extending. Rather than allow this to happen, do not lower your body as far and support yourself by holding onto a chair to take some of your body-weight.

Exercise 91	Anterior chest and shoulders

Starting position and instructions

Standing side on to a wall, place your right hand on the wall at shoulder height. Keeping your right arm straight, turn your feet to the left and rotate your body to the left, feeling the stretch across the front of your right shoulder. This movement stretches the anterior deltoid, pectoral and biceps muscles.

Variations

Altering the height of the hand on the wall will vary the site of the stretch.

Points to note

Because of the momentum involved in this exercise, the trunk twist must be slow and controlled at all times.

Exercise 92	Shoulder flexors

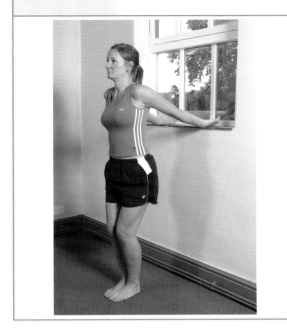

Exercise 93	External shoulder rotation – using a stick

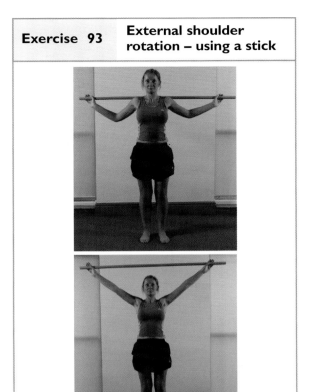

Starting position and instructions

Keeping your arms straight, extend them behind you and place the back of your hands on a high table. Maintaining correct body alignment, bend your knees to lower your body, pressing your shoulders into further extension. This movement stretches the anterior deltoid, pectoral and biceps muscles.

Variations

Putting your hands closer together or further apart changes the muscle emphasis of the exercise.

Points to note

In cases of shoulder dislocation, this exercise should not be used: as the arm is forced back into extension, the ball of the shoulder (head of the humerus) moves forwards in the joint, stressing the anterior structures.

Starting position and instructions

Grip a bar above your head. Lower your arms so that the bar passes behind your neck, hold the position and then release. This movement stretches the medial rotators of the shoulder (subscapularis, deltoid, latissimus dorsi and pectoralis major).

Variations

A towel can be used instead of the bar, provided that you keep the towel taut.

Points to note

Asymmetry in rotation is common, so one arm may be able to drop lower than the other.

Exercise 94	Combined shoulder rotation – using a towel

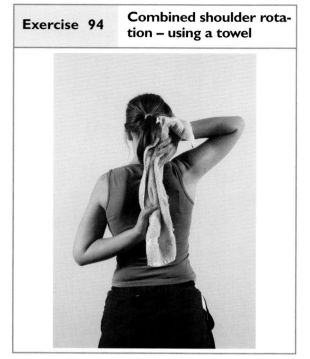

Starting position and instructions

Grasp a towel behind your back with your right arm placed behind your neck and your left arm in the small of your back. Move your arms up and down to lift and lower the towel vertically.

Variations

A broom handle can be used instead of the towel, or, if you are very flexible, you may be able to grasp your hands together. If you perform the exercise sitting or kneeling on the floor, bending the trunk slightly will increase the intensity of the stretch by pressing the lower arm further backwards.

Points to note

Asymmetry in shoulder rotation is common, so the range of motion may differ when the arm placement changes.

Exercise 95	Forearm flexors

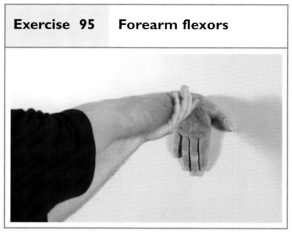

Starting position and instructions

Place your right hand flat against a wall with your fingers pointing to the floor and your right arm straight. Hold your right elbow locked using your left hand. Lean your body-weight forwards, pressing the heel of your right hand into the wall.

Variations

Placing your hand higher up the wall will increase the stretch.

Points to note

Releasing the elbow even very slightly will make the stretch less effective.

Exercise 96	Thumb flexors and abductors

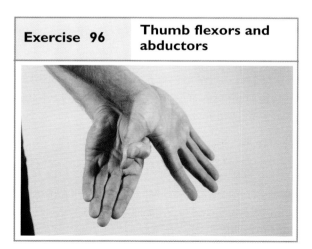

Starting position and instructions

Place your right hand palm up on a table with your thumb extended. With your left hand, grip your right thumb from beneath and pull your thumb into extension and abduction.

Variations

Altering the exact position of the thumb will vary the site of the stretch.

Points to note

Because of the leverage involved in this stretch, the force applied should be slow and continuous rather than sudden.

Starting position and instructions

This is a classic yoga pose called *Vrksasana* or the Tree. Stand with your feet hip width apart. Shift your body-weight to the left to take the weight off your right leg. Bend your right leg at the hip and knee and place the sole of your right foot as far up your inner left leg as possible, with your toes pointing downwards. Press the right knee backwards until it is in line with your body. Hold the posture for 30–60 seconds, breathing normally.

Variations

First you can perform the movement while holding onto a fixed point such as a wall bar or a piece of gym apparatus. Support yourself with the hand opposite to the leg you are lifting; use your left hand when your are lifting your right leg, for example. Second, you can make the movement easier by not lifting your leg as high, placing your foot on your ankle, shin, or below the knee rather than above it.

Points to note

There is a tendency for the foot to slip in this movement. This can be counteracted by pressing the foot firmly in towards the knee and, at the same time, firmly straightening the straight leg and pressing it slightly into adduction so that the leg presses against the knee.

Exercise 97   The Tree

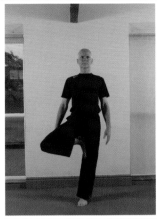

(a)

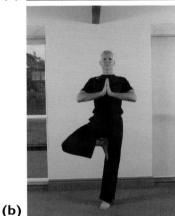

(b)

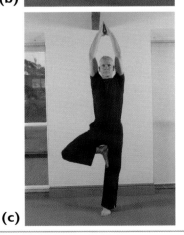

(c)

PARTNER STRETCHES

10

Partner stretches are useful because they enable you to relax while your partner supplies the force for the stretch. In addition, working with a partner or personal trainer can boost motivation. However, there is one thing you should be careful of with partner stretches. When you perform a stretch by yourself, the sensation you feel in the muscles is used to limit the force that you apply. In short, if it hurts, you stop. With partner stretches, however, your partner cannot feel your pain, so you must keep him or her informed throughout the stretch about exactly how the exercise feels.

A physiotherapist or experienced personal trainer will be able to feel tissue tension, that is the feel of the tissue as it is stretched. Normally when you stretch a muscle the feeling is one of elasticity. As the stretch continues, the elasticity also continues but is not as strong, a little like the difference between stretching a thick elastic band and then stretching a thinner one. When you stretch the thigh to the chest, however, the tissue tension feels soft. This is because when you are quite flexible, the thigh presses against the pelvis and chest, compressing the thick thigh muscles. The difference in the feel of tissue tension, therefore, is between muscle stretch and general soft tissue compression. For example, when stretching the shoulder to rotation, the tissue tension feels slightly elastic, but is firmer than the feel of a general muscle stretch. This is because in rotation the shoulder ligaments and joint capsule are also being stretched instead of just the shoulder muscles. However, when stretching your elbow to extension (out straight), the tissue tension is hard. This is due to bone hitting bone at the back of the elbow. Clearly, bone cannot be stretched, so when the tissue tension feel is hard, a personal trainer will ease off as they know that no further stretch is possible.

There are both advantages and disadvantages of partner work. On the plus side, motivation is better, but on the minus side, the exercise is less controlled because two people are involved. Therefore, when practising partner stretches a stable starting position must be chosen to avoid either person falling and violently increasing the stretch. The two partners act as one unit, so their combined mass has a single base of support and a single line of gravity (*see* chapter 1), with the base of support being larger than it would be for a single person. The person applying the stretch must move into a comfortable position that they can easily maintain, rather than moving into an awkward position that places them off balance so that they have to continuously readjust their position.

If partner activities are used in a group exercise situation, they must be practised under the supervision of an experienced and skilled instructor. Close supervision of individuals in the group is essential, especially when dealing with young or inexperienced individuals. When teaching partner work to adolescents, they should be matched for body size and degree of flexibility.

> **Key point**: Partner stretches introduce variety to training and are good for motivation. The danger of overstretching is ever present, however, so communication between partners is essential.

Exercise 98	**Hip flexors – supine lying**

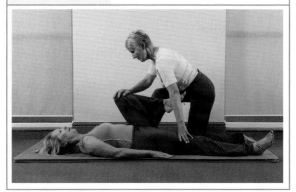

Starting position and instructions

Lie on the floor with your right hip and knee flexed. Your partner half kneels at your right hip. With their right hand they hold your left leg on the floor, and with their left hand they press your right leg into further hip flexion. This movement stretches the rectus femoris and iliopsoas of the lower leg, and the gluteals of the upper leg.

Variations

For those who experience pain in their knee, the partner's hand should be positioned on the under side of the knee.

Points to note

Most individuals are asymmetrical, so one leg may appear less flexible than the other.

Exercise 99	**Hip adductors – stride sitting**

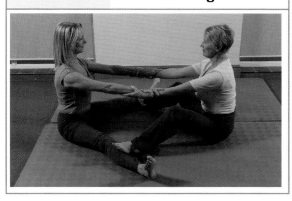

Starting position and instructions

Sit on the floor with your hips abducted. Your partner sits in front of you and places their stockinged feet on your inner shins. Link arms, and your partner presses your legs apart while pulling your trunk forwards. Hinge at the hips, keeping your spine aligned throughout the action.

Variations

Instead of pulling arm to arm, your partner can place a towel around your waist and pull your trunk forwards by pulling on the towel. This reduces the leverage on the spine.

Points to note

There must be equal pressure between pressing with the feet and pulling on the trunk to increase flexibility. The aim of the trunk pull is simply to encourage pelvic tilt, moving the buttocks (ischial tuberosity) backwards in relation to the knee. When trunk flexion occurs, the stretch has moved from the adductors to the trunk tissues.

Exercise 100	Hip adductors – sitting back to back

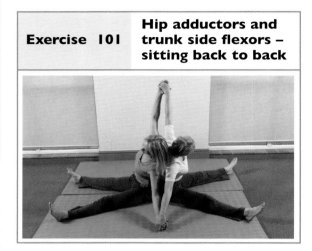

Exercise 101	Hip adductors and trunk side flexors – sitting back to back

Starting position and instructions

Sit on the floor with your legs as far apart as possible. Your partner sits in the same position with their back to you. Sit close together with your tail bones touching. Lean forwards and place your hands on the ground, trying to bend from your waist only. At the same time, your partner reaches overhead with both arms and leans back onto you, extending their spine as you flex forwards. Hold the stretch position for 20–30 seconds and then reverse, reaching overhead and arching your back over your partner.

Variations

If you find that your back is bending too much, place 3–4 yoga blocks in front of you and lean your elbows on the blocks rather than placing your hands on the floor. Try to emphasise the movement of the hips by performing a forward (anterior) tilt of your pelvis and maintaining the hollow in the small of your back.

Points to note

As you are taking the weight of your partner's trunk on your own, there is a tendency for you to flex your spine excessively if your hips are very tight. If this occurs, the exercise is not suitable for

you. Some bending (flexion) of the spine may occur, which should be balanced by straightening your spine (extension) as you stretch over your partner.

Starting position and instructions

Sit back to back with your partner and abduct your hips into a stretched stride position. Link hands and lean to the right, bending your right arm and placing your forearm on the ground, pulling your partner to their left. Maintain this side-leaning position and reach your left arm overhead and to the right side, pulling your partner's right arm to the left as you do so. Maintain the position for 20–30 seconds and then reverse the movement, stretching to your left side.

Variations

Rather than holding hands with your partner, you can hold a stick or broom handle between you in an overhead grip. As you lean to the side, however, you will not be able to take your weight through your forearms, so be careful not to stretch too far.

Points to note

By gripping each others hands, you avoid the tendency to bend forwards. However, you must make sure first, that you are both the same size so that your arm length matches, and second that one person does not pull excessively as you bend to the side.

Exercise 102	Hip abductors – side lying (Ober position)

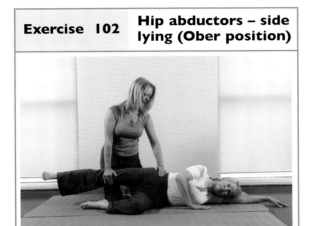

Starting position and instructions

Lie on a bench or the floor on your left-hand side; your partner kneels behind you at waist level. Your partner abducts and extends your right leg with their lower arm while fixing your pelvis with their upper arm. Keeping the pelvis stable (avoiding any side tilt) and pressing your right leg down into adduction stretches the abductors.

Variations

Flexing the leg will emphasise the posterior portion of the gluteus medius.

Points to note

Allowing even a small amount of pelvic movement will completely release the stretch in this exercise. You will only feel the stretch if you have tightness in the hip abductors of the upper leg.

Exercise 103	Hip rotation – lying

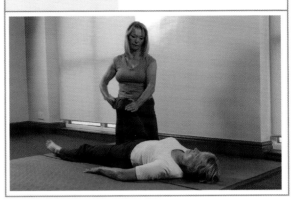

Starting position and instructions

Lie on the floor on your back with your partner kneeling at your right-hand side by your waist. Your partner flexes your right knee and hip and presses it inwards and outwards, encouraging rotation at the hip. This movement stretches the medial and lateral rotators of the hip.

Variations

Altering the angle of hip flexion will vary the stress on the hip rotators.

Points to note

This exercise places stress on the pelvic joints, so it must be used with caution following pregnancy.

Exercise 104	Hamstrings – lying on back

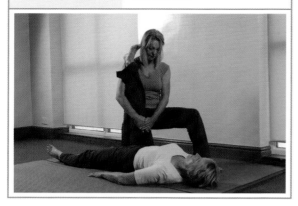

Starting position and instructions

Lie on the floor with your legs straight. Your partner half kneels at your right hip and lifts your right leg, placing their hand over your knee to keep the leg straight. Your leg rests on your partner's shoulder and they lunge forwards, pressing your leg into further flexion at the hip.

Variations

Place a small pad on your partner's shoulder and a small rolled towel under your back to make the position more comfortable.

Points to note

This exercise is most effective when used with PNF techniques. When locking the leg out straight, make sure that the pressure is not placed directly over the kneecap. Cup your hand and place it around, but not directly on top of, your partner's knee.

Exercise 105	Hamstrings – standing (wall support)

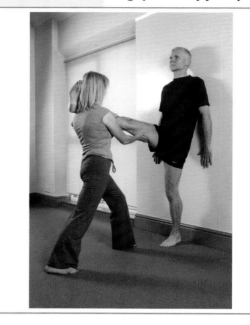

Starting position and instructions

Stand with your back to a wall; your partner stands facing you in a lunge stance, knees slightly bent. Place your right leg on your partner's right shoulder and take hold of their arms, keeping your leg straight. Your partner gradually straightens their legs, pressing your right leg into further flexion.

Variations

If you are extremely flexible, your partner can place their hands together and hold your foot as they press your hip into further flexion above their shoulder. If you are less flexible, your partner can cup their hands around your leg and lift it to the level of their waist.

Points to note

Stability is important, so if you find you are unstable during this exercise, hold on to the wall.

Exercise 106	Gastrocnemius in lying

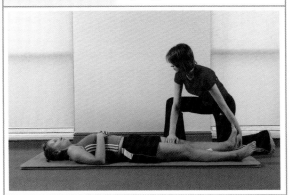

Exercise 107	Flat back hamstring stretch – the 'table top'

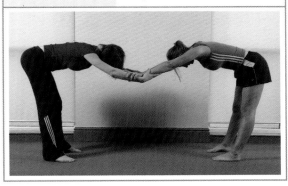

Starting position and instructions

Lie on the floor with partner half kneeling at your shins. Your partner places a folded towel beneath your right calf and cups their hand around your right heel. Get your partner to lunge forwards, pressing their forearm against your foot to push your foot into dorsiflexion (toes upwards).

Variations

Placing the folded towel beneath your knee, flex the knee throwing the stress from the long calf muscle (gastrocnemius) to the short calf muscle (soleus).

Points to note

The calf and Achilles are very powerful and often very tight. It is essential that your partner places the stretch on using their body-weight rather than simply their hands. Using only the hands places considerable stress on the hand and finger joints.

Starting position and instructions

Stand facing your partner about half a body length apart with your feet hip width apart and your legs straight. Your partner should have their feet twice hip width apart and their knees slightly bent (soft). Hold hands with your partner and, keeping your trunk very straight, bend forwards at the hips and reach your arms out to rest at the level of your partners hips. Your partner takes the weight of your upper body as you do so, holding their hands close to their hips.

Variations

You can also perform this exercise by both leaning forwards. In this case, begin by standing a full body length apart and lean forwards slowly until you are able to hold hands. At the end of the movement, your upper bodies and arms should be completely flat and in line.

Points to note

The aim of this movement is to place the stretch on the hamstrings by tilting the pelvis forwards and keeping the spine straight or even slightly hollow in the lumbar spine (lumbar lordosis maintained). To facilitate this, pull your abdomen in and slightly brace your shoulders while pressing your chest outwards (thoracic extension). With the

149

first movement, some of your body-weight is taken by your partner. In the variation, you both support your own full weight and use each other purely for balance, therefore emphasising strength as well as stretch.

Exercise 108	Sit and reach – back to back

Starting position and instructions

Sit on the floor back to back with your partner with your tailbones touching and your legs out straight. Lean forwards towards your toes, supporting your body-weight by resting your forearms on your thighs. At the same time, your partner reaches overhead with both arms and leans back onto you. Allow the overpressure of your partners weight to press you further forwards, keeping your back as straight as possible.

Variations

To place less overload on the stretch, your partner can keep their arms by their sides rather than reaching overhead.

Points to note

This stretch relies on you both having approximately the same upper-body length. If one of you is shorter, they can sit on one or two yoga blocks to bring your shoulders up to the same

height. Also, if one person is heavier than the other, they will apply greater pressure simply through their body-weight. Make sure, therefore, that you are weight-matched with your partner.

Exercise 109	Lower back flexion – sitting

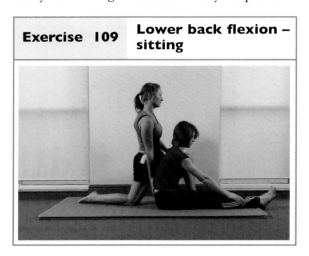

Starting position and instructions

Sit on a mat with your knees loosely bent and wider than hip width apart. Your partner kneels behind you. Bend forwards from the hips, placing your hands on the floor for support. At the end of the movement, your partner places overload on your lower back to increase the stretch.

Variations

Straightening the legs slightly throws extra stress on the hamstring muscles. Sitting with a folded towel or yoga block under your sitting bones (ischial tuberosities) tilts your pelvis forwards and assists alignment.

Points to note

The aim of this movement is to tilt the pelvis forwards with minimal spinal flexion. Overpressure must be placed on the lumbar spine and not between the shoulder blades. If your partner presses too high up, the tendency is to increase flexion of the thoracic spine rather than increasing the forward pelvic tilt.

Exercise 110	Rectus femoris – prone

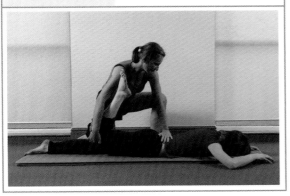

Exercise 111	Anterior chest and shoulders – prone

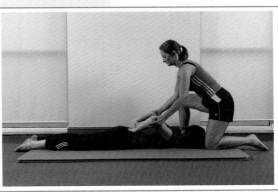

Starting position and instructions

Lie on the floor on your front and bend your right knee. Your partner half kneels at your right hip and places one hand in the small of your back and the other beneath your right knee. Your right foot rests on your partner's shoulder. By leaning forwards, your partner presses your right leg into extension at the hip and flexion at the knee while preventing any lumbar movement.

Variations

Increasing the amount of hip extension will emphasise the upper portion of the muscle; reducing hip extension but increasing knee flexion targets the lower portion.

Points to note

Abduction of the hip should be avoided during this exercise as it releases some of the stretch from the rectus femoris.

Starting position and instructions

Lie on the floor on your front with both hands in the small of your back. Your partner kneels at your head. Grasping your outer elbows, your partner leans back to pull your arms inwards and upwards. This movement stretches the anterior deltoid, pectoral and biceps muscles.

Variations

Pressing the elbows closer together, or leaving them further apart, will alter the exact site of the stretch.

Points to note

As with all partner stretches, the subject receiving the stretch must give feedback to lead the movement at all times. As the arm is pulled back (extension), the ball of the shoulder socket (head of the humerus) moves forwards. If you have had a shoulder dislocation, this movement should not be practised, as it can overstretch the already lax anterior structures of the joint.

DYNAMIC STRETCHES

11

Guidelines for dynamic stretching

We saw in chapter 4 that dynamic stretching is simply stretching with movement. It is similar to ballistic stretching as it uses the speed of the body's movement to assist the stretch (as opposed to static stretching, which uses no movement), but dynamic stretching does not involve the bouncing for which ballistic stretching is famous. Dynamic stretching usually uses the body's full range of motion at either single or multiple joints and makes the stretch more functional, as it involves a combination of several different fitness components including stretching, muscle contraction, muscle control and movement rehearsal (skill and timing). The action is therefore specific to the movement patterns involved in sport or daily living, and as such closely follows the *specificity principles* outlined on page 51.

> **Key point**: Dynamic stretching uses movement patterns rather than static stretches and therefore can be highly specific to a sports action.

All dynamic stretching exercises should be performed after a warm-up of a sufficient intensity to induce light sweating, such as a brisk walk, static cycling or a gentle jog. Once you are warm, static stretches relevant to the dynamic movement to be used should be practised. For example, an arm swing dynamic stretch should be preceded by overhead reaching. The aim is to take the limb through the full range of motion used in the dynamic stretch.

Initially, all dynamic stretches should be performed while stationary (also called 'in place') and once the exercise is familiar the movement can be performed while moving. Using an arm swing action as an example again, the movement is performed for 5–10 repetitions while standing still. After a brief (30-second) rest, the movement is repeated while walking. This additional movement serves to develop coordination, as you will not be able to simply focus your attention on the arm action alone. Table 11.1 summarises these guidelines.

Combined movements

In everyday movements, and especially in sport, we rarely perform 'pure' actions such as flexion or extension. These movements are said to be 'single plane' actions as they occur in only one of the three body planes (*see* page 13). In reality, we normally combine the three movement planes and perform actions such as flexion with abduction and rotation. This combination of movements is more demanding in terms of coordination, and so must be practised gradually.

Leg actions such as kicking combine actions across the body: flexion with adduction, followed by extension with abduction. In each case

Table 11.1	Guidelines for the practice of dynamic stretching exercises

- Begin with a warm-up sufficient to induce mild sweating
- Perform static stretching matched to the bodypart and range of motion to be used in dynamic stretching
- Perform the dynamic stretch in a slow controlled manner
- Progress the speed of movement gradually until it matches that to be used in sport
- Perform the dynamic stretch while standing still
- Progress to walking activities

the movements may also be combined with medial or lateral rotation. Throwing actions again combine cross-body actions (flexion and adduction) beginning with a 'wind-up' phase of abduction and extension.

Both throwing and kicking will also use trunk actions. For example, a wind-up for a throw will use trunk rotation, lateral flexion and extension towards the extended arm, followed by trunk rotation, lateral flexion and flexion to follow the throwing arm as it goes forwards in front of the body. A kicking action in football will often combine hip flexion and adduction with medial rotation to strike the ball with the inside of the foot. A round house kick in martial arts combines trunk rotation with hip flexion, abduction and medial rotation to strike the target with the front of the foot or shin.

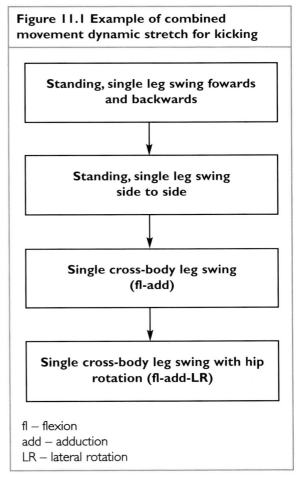

Figure 11.1 Example of combined movement dynamic stretch for kicking

Standing, single leg swing fowards and backwards

↓

Standing, single leg swing side to side

↓

Single cross-body leg swing (fl-add)

↓

Single cross-body leg swing with hip rotation (fl-add-LR)

fl – flexion
add – adduction
LR – lateral rotation

As these actions are complex, they are best trained by performing the actual sport technique but at a lower level and to repetition. For example, the football kick would be performed slowly at a low level, gradually building up speed and intensity as the player progresses. An example of progression to full kicking is shown in figure 11.1.

Exercise 112	Arm swing – forwards

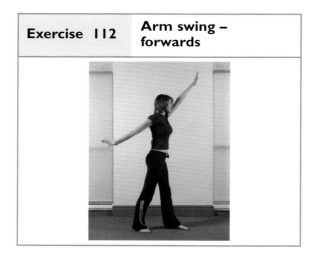

Exercise 113	Arm swing – sideways

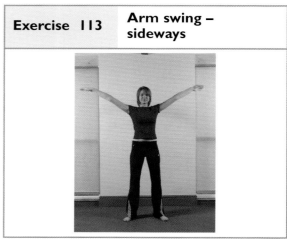

Starting position and instructions

Stand with your feet shoulder width apart and knees slightly bent (soft). Swing the right arm upwards and forwards to shoulder level, then allow it to travel back behind the bodyline by 1–2 hand breaths. Pause, and then repeat using the left arm. Once you are confident with the movement, cut out the pause between the movements and practise alternate arm swings as a single continuous motion.

Variations

Both arms can be swung together rather than alternately. However, make sure that you maintain low back alignment as the arms are swung forwards. Do not allow the lower back to hollow excessively (hyperextend) as the arms are taken overhead.

Points to note

The range of motion of the movement should increase progressively. At first, only swing the arm to shoulder level, and with each repetition gradually increase the range of motion until the arm is taken overhead. The rate of progression will be dictated by your fitness level and shoulder flexibility.

Starting position and instructions

Stand with your feet just wider than shoulder width apart and your knees slightly bent (soft). Swing both arms out to the side, allowing the arm to turn (rotate) naturally so that the thumb points towards the ceiling. Lengthen the arm, avoiding any tendency to shrug your shoulders.

Variations

If you have had a shoulder problem, sideways movements (abduction) can be painful. If this applies to you, limit the movement of this stretch by keeping the arm below shoulder level. If you experience no pain and have practised static stretching without problems, slowly increase the range of motion until you can reach overhead and, eventually, touch your hands together.

Points to note

Do not allow your lower back to hollow excessively (hyperextend) as the arms are taken overhead. Maintain your back alignment by tightening your abdominal muscles slightly to increase your core stability.

Exercise 114	Arm rotation – alternate

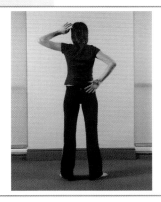

Exercise 115	Flexion/extension – standing

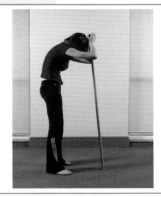

Starting position and instructions

Stand with your feet shoulder width apart and your knees slightly bent (soft). Take your right arm overhead and touch the back of your head with your right hand. Now, take your left hand backwards and place it behind the small of your back. Reverse the movement, alternating between arms. Gradually speed the movement up so that the exercise becomes a smooth, continuous action.

Variations

If you are unable to take your hand behind your head or back, limit the movement by touching only your ear and the outside of your hip. Gradually increase your range of motion using static stretching before you progress the range of the dynamic stretch.

Points to note

Maintain your alignment throughout the movement. As you reach your arm behind your back, do not allow your shoulder to move forwards. As you reach behind your neck, do not hollow your back.

Starting position and instructions

Stand with your knees hip width apart and slightly bent (soft). Hold on to a vertical pole with your arms horizontal for balance. Tilt your pelvis backwards, round your shoulders and flex your spine. Pause in this flexed position, then tilt your pelvis forwards, brace your shoulders and extend your spine. Gradually speed up the movement until you are performing a single smooth action.

Variations

When you are confident with the movement, you can dispense with the stick. When you do this, the exercise works your sense of balance (proprioception) harder. However, make sure that you avoid too much body sway when you do this.

Points to note

Depending on your posture type (*see* pages 78–81) you may find either flexion or extension easier. If this is the case, do not force the stiff movement with dynamic stretching. Instead, develop your flexibility using static stretching, and then maintain it with dynamic stretching.

Exercise 116   Flexion/extension – kneeling

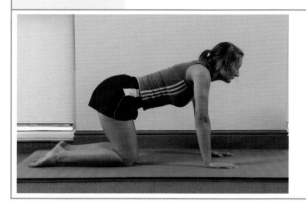 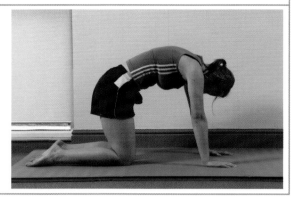

Starting position and instructions

Kneel down on all fours with your knees hip width apart and your hands shoulder width apart. Your knees should be directly below your hips and your hands directly below your shoulders. Round (flex) your spine and tuck your tail under (posterior pelvic tilt). Pause in this position, then arch (extend) your spine and point your tail to the ceiling (anterior pelvic tilt). Build the action into a single smooth movement.

Variations

You can include hip flexion and extension in this action: as you round your spine, draw your right knee towards your forehead. As you arch your spine, straighten your right leg and take it slightly upwards. Repeat the movement with the other leg.

Points to note

If you use the leg variation, make sure that you control the actions throughout, cutting down the momentum of the moving leg. If the leg moves too quickly, the spine will be forced to flex and extend at the end of each sequence by the movement of the leg. This can introduce dangerous loading forces to the lumbar vertebrae (low back bones) in particular.

Exercise 117	Lateral flexion – standing

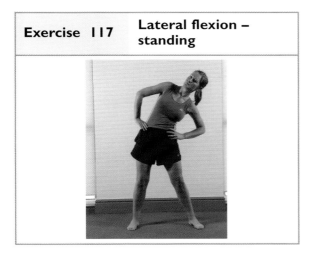

Starting position and instructions

Stand with your feet 1½ times shoulder width apart and place your hands on your hips. Bend to the right, taking your weight on your right arm. Stand up straight again and then bend to the left, taking your weight on your left arm.

Variations

Once you are confident with the movement, release your arms and perform the action with your arms by your sides. This increases the work of the trunk muscles as they now have to support your full body-weight. Finally, you can increase the stretch by reaching overhead. As you bend to the left, reach overhead (and slightly to the left) with your right hand. Reverse the action using the left hand as you bend to the right.

Points to note

It is common to have some asymmetry, with this movement as many people have a greater degree of flexion to one side than the other. If this is the case, develop your flexibility using the supported side bend (hands on your hips) rather than reaching overhead. Once you have an equal range of motion on both sides, you can progress to the overhead reach action.

Exercise 118	Rotation – standing

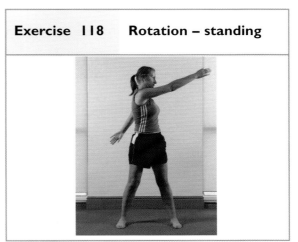

Starting position and instructions

Stand with your feet shoulder width apart and your knees slightly bent (soft). Your arms should be held slightly away from your body. Turn your body to the left, bringing your right arm round in front of you and pointing your hand to the left. At the same time, take your left hand behind you, pointing your hand to the right. Reverse the action.

Variations

You can reduce the forces on the spine by performing the action with your hands on your hips. In this case, the elbows lead the movement and some of your body-weight is taken through your hips.

Points to note

Make sure that your arms lead the movement, but do not allow them to swing vigorously to force you further into rotation.

Exercise 119   Rotation – lying

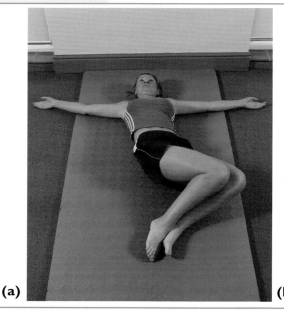

(a)

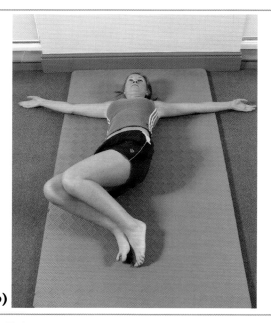

(b)

Starting position and instructions

Lie on your back with your knees bent and feet flat. Keep your arms out to your sides at an angle of 45 degrees to your body. Allow your knees to slowly lower to one side, twisting your trunk as they do so. Pause in the lower position as your knee touches the mat and then pull your leg back up. Repeat to each side.

Variations

If you lift your feet up from the mat so that your knees are directly above your hips, the emphasis is changed to strength throughout the move-ment. Rather than placing your arms on the mat to support your upper body, you can move your arms in the opposite direction to your legs (knees to the right, arms to the left), which places a greater stretch on the thoracic spine.

Points to note

As the knee is lowered on to the mat, ensure that you keep the action under control. Do not allow your knees to drop, forcing your spine into a rotation range that may be inappropriate. If you find the rotation range too great, allow your knees to lower onto a cushion or block rather than all the way down on to the mat.

Exercise 120   Cervical rotation

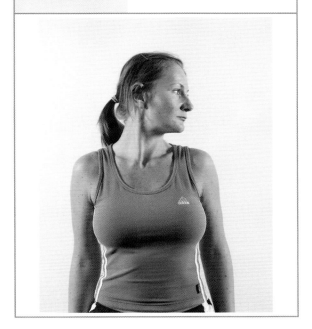

Starting position and instructions

Sit on a chair or gym bench with your spine correctly aligned. Sit up tall and draw your chin in slightly. Relax your shoulders and avoid the tendency to shrug them. Loosely fold your arms on your lap to support their weight and assist in shoulder relaxation. Keep your shoulders square, look to your right as far as is comfortable, pause in this rotated position and then look to your left. Repeat the action five times, making sure that you pause at each side to avoid feeling dizzy. With each repetition, try to gradually increase your range of motion until your chin passes over your collarbone (clavicle).

Variations

As you twist, you may find that your neck moves into flexion or extension; this means that the rotation movement is not a single pure movement, but is combined with flexion/extension. To avoid this, hold a stick or ruler in front of you just below your nose. As you practise the movement, make sure that your nose does not move away from the ruler (neck extension) or touch the ruler (neck flexion).

Points to note

It is common to suffer asymmetry (where one side of the body is different from the other) in the cervical spine. If you notice that the rotation to one side is less than that to the other side, do not force the movement on the stiff side.

Exercise 121   Leg swing – sideways

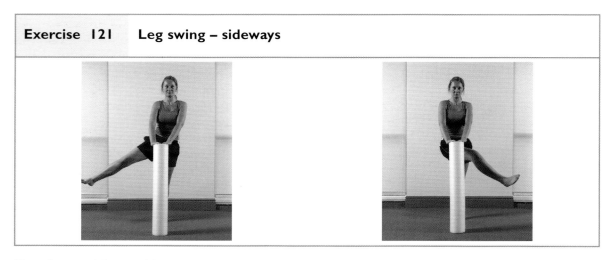

Starting position and instructions

Stand facing a piece of gym equipment with your feet hip width apart. Hold on to the apparatus with both hands. Shift your pelvis to the left to take your whole weight onto your left leg and unload your right. Swing your right leg out to the side and then inwards and in front of the left leg (abduction and adduction). Start by swinging outwards to shin level, then knee level and finally hip level. As you swing your leg, do not allow your trunk to twist.

Variations

Pointing your toes to the ceiling combines hip abduction with lateral rotation. Pointing the your heel to the ceiling (toes to the floor) combines abduction with medial rotation. Use both actions to balance your training programme unless your medial rotators are especially long, in which case the lateral rotation movement alone should be emphasised.

Points to note

In order to unload the swinging leg, you must transfer your body-weight over the other (weight-bearing) leg. This should be achieved by shifting the pelvis over the weight-bearing leg. However, if you lack hip control and hip stability,

you may find that you simply tip your spine sideways (lateral flexion of the trunk). Try to avoid this action by keeping your spine upright and your pelvis level.

Exercise 122   Leg swing – forwards and backwards

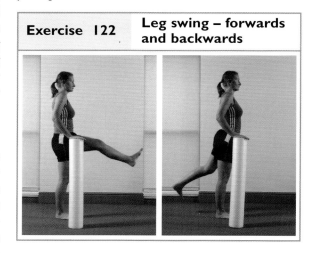

Starting position and instructions

Stand with your feet shoulder width apart. Hold on to a bar or the frame of a piece of gym apparatus at your right side for balance. Swing your left leg forwards and upwards into flexion, first to shin level, then to waist level and eventually to chest level. Progress the range of motion as you feel comfortable, being careful not to overstretch.

As the limb goes backwards, maintain your low back alignment; do not allow your back to hollow excessively (hyperextend).

Variations

Keeping the leg straight places the stretch on the single joint hip flexors (iliopsoas) and the extensors. Allowing the knee to bend as though kicking the backside will stretch the rectus femoris as well.

Points to note

Ensure, therefore, that the action is controlled throughout the whole range of movement. Do not allow the momentum to pull you into a range that you would not usually use.

Exercise 123	Knee to elbow

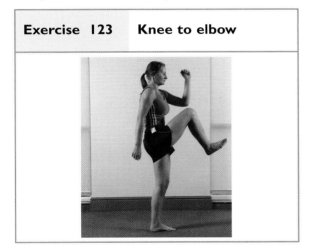

Starting position and instructions

Stand with your feet shoulder width apart and your arms held slightly abducted with your forearms horizontal. Bring your right knee up to touch your right elbow, lower the leg and then repeat, this time bringing your left knee to your left elbow.

Variations

You can also use a diagonal pattern, taking the right knee to the left elbow and vice versa. The movement can be progressed to a knee-to-elbow walk by placing the foot forwards rather than directly downwards and moving along in a high-knee walk.

Points to note

Make sure that you pull your knee up to your elbow rather than bending forwards and taking your elbow down to your knee. Aim to keep your trunk upright and your spine vertical throughout the exercise.

Exercise 124	Lunge walk

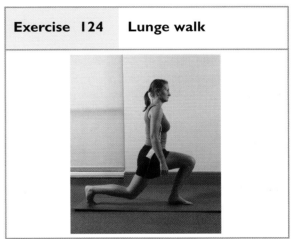

Starting position and instructions

Stand with your feet shoulder width apart and your hands by your sides. Step forwards with your right leg in a lunging action, placing your foot flat on the floor. Aim to have your knee pass beyond your foot and your thigh horizontal. Step back so that your feet are again shoulder width apart and repeat the movement with your left leg. Once you have performed five repetitions on each leg, rest for 30–60 seconds. Then step forwards with your right leg into a lunge, press yourself back up again and then step forwards with the left, aiming to move along in a deep 'walking' action.

Variations

Initially, you perform the lunge walk with your arms by your sides. However, the balance of the movement is made easier if you extend your arms out sideways in a 'T' position. If you find the lunge is too hard on your legs, place one hand on the thigh of the forward lunging leg and press on it to bring yourself back up to standing.

Points to note

The downward movement of the lunge must be controlled; take care not to 'fall' into the position. In addition, make sure that you keep your trunk upright, avoiding the temptation to lead forwards by flexing the trunk on the hip. Fix your eyes on a distant point to help you with this.

muscles to allow free movement of your heels. Pull your feet towards you, then point them away from you.

Variations

This exercise can also be performed by hooking an exercise band around the ball of your feet. Allow the band to pull your feet upwards (dorsiflexion), then point your toes against the resistance of the band. You can perform the stretch one leg at a time if this feels more comfortable. Hooking the band around your toes rather than the ball of your foot will also place the stretch on the deep toe flexors as well as the calf.

Exercise 125	**Calf stretch – with band**

Starting position and instructions

Sit on a mat with your legs straight out in front of you. Place a rolled towel beneath your calf

Points to note

There are two main calf muscles: the soleus, which acts over the ankle alone; and the gastrocnemius, which acts over both the ankle and the knee. To target the gastrocnemius muscle (the larger of the two), perform the action with your knees straight. To work the soleus muscle, perform the movement with your knees slightly bent.

Variations

Placing your back leg further back will increase the intensity of the stretch; taking your leg further forwards will reduce it. You can emphasise the power aspect of this movement rather than

Exercise 126	Calf stretch – sprint start

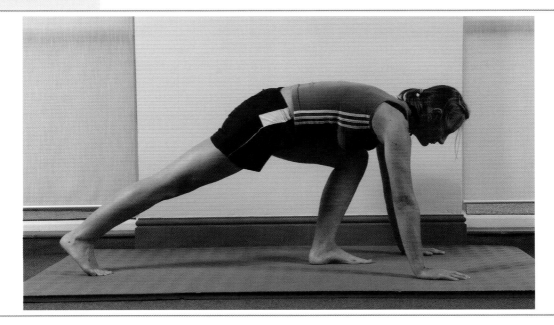

Starting position and instructions

Stand in a lunge position with your right leg back and your left leg forwards, with your weight over your front leg. Place the toes of your back foot on the ground and gradually take your weight backwards, forcing your heel onto the ground as you do so. Pause, then use the calf strength of your back leg to 'flick' you forwards as though exploding out of the blocks from a sprint start. Repeat the exercise five times with the right leg back, then reverse the movement.

the stretch by taking more weight on to your back leg and jumping slightly as you flick yourself forwards.

Points to note

Make sure that you build the range of motion progressively. Start with your feet quite close together and gradually move your back leg further backwards as your confidence in the movement grows.

STRETCHING THE NERVES

12

Stretching exercises are generally said to effect the muscles, with less effect on the joint tissues. However, an important structure that may be affected when performing stretching exercises is the nervous system.

Any exercise that moves a limb will have effects on the nerves as well as the muscles, and these effects must be considered when giving stretching exercises. As a limb is bent or straightened, the nerves must adapt. With elbow flexion, for example, the ulnar nerve is stretched while the radial and median nerves are shortened. In fact, from fully bending the elbow and wrist to fully straightening them, nerves can change their length by as much as 20 per cent. Any stretching exercise we perform will have effects on the nerves and, through them, on other tissues seemingly unconnected to the body-part we are using.

> **Key point**: In normal movements, nerves may stretch (lengthen) by up to 20 per cent.

Structure of the nervous system

The nervous system can be visualised as an 'H' turned on its side, with the central bar of the 'H' being the spinal cord and the crossbars the nerves to the arms and legs. This structure is often divided into the central nervous system (CNS), consisting of the brain and spinal cord, and the peripheral nervous system, consisting of the nerves in the legs and arms. However, this division is misleading, because structurally many of the tissues within the nervous system are connected with each other, and the chemical reactions and electrical impulses within the nervous system travel its entire length. The nervous system can, therefore, be considered as a 'continuous tissue tract', a little like a single piece of string looping through the spine and limbs. Any tension (pulling) on one part will be transmitted throughout the whole structure and will have effects at points distant to the original site of disruption.

There are two types of nerve cells in nervous tissue: those that carry electrical nerve impulses (neurons), and those that protect and support the delicate conducting structures of the nervous system (neuroglial cells). In the limbs, the peripheral nervous system is made up of neurons, which have a cell body and long arms stretching out into the limb (*see* fig 12.1). The cell body is located close to the spine, with the cell's arm stretching the whole length of the limb. For example, a single nerve cell may stretch from the lumbar spine along the whole length of the leg to the big toe! The cell's arm (axon) is covered with an insulating material called myelin, which is produced from the neuroglial cells. The structure of the axon can be compared to an electrical cable of copper wire covered with insulating rubber. The nerve cells are grouped into bundles (fascicles) and the bundles are covered by a variety of membranes, the innermost being the endoneurium.

Figure 12.1 Structure of a nerve cell

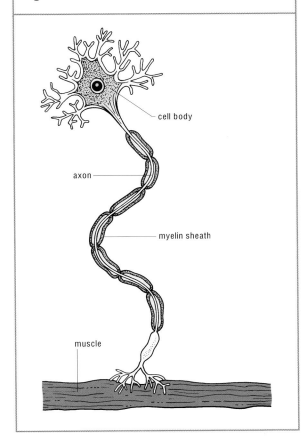

cell body

axon

myelin sheath

muscle

exposed to stress from certain movements and back injuries.

> **Key point:** The nerves of the limbs (arms and legs) join the spinal cord via the nerve roots.

Attached alongside the spinal cord is the autonomic nervous system (part of the peripheral nervous system and consisting of sympathetic and parasympathetic parts), which provides the nervous control of the internal body environment, regulating, for example, heart rate and blood pressure. In addition, it controls aspects of the skin such as sweating and skin blood flow. Involvement of the autonomic nervous system in injury may, for example, cause whiteness in the skin with feelings of hot and cold, and sweating.

Biomechanics of the nervous system

When nerves are stretched, they can do only one of two things: they can lengthen or 'give', or they can *develop tension*. Tension development is in the form of compression of the tissues and fluids contained in the nerve sheaths.

Movement of the nervous system may occur as a whole (gross movement), as in the case of a nerve sliding through a bony tunnel on the outside of the elbow. This movement may also be quite large: in the case of the spinal cord moving from full extension to full flexion, the cord can lengthen by nearly 10 cm, most of the movement being in the cervical and lumbar regions with little movement in the thoracic spine. With traction used by physiotherapists, a 5 kg stretching force can elongate the cervical spine by 10 mm and therefore stretch the spinal cord. Compression caused by carrying heavy weights will similarly compress the spine.

In the central nervous system, the brain connects to the spinal cord at the base of the skull, and from the cord 'nerve roots' arise at 'T' junctions.

Several nerve roots may come together to form a peripheral nerve travelling into the limbs. The cord, nerve root and peripheral nerve each have a protective covering, but that of the nerve root is different from the other two structures. In addition, the point at which the nerve root leaves the spinal cord is very close to the vertebral bones themselves, so the space is restricted. The combination of restricted space and poorer protection leaves the nerve root

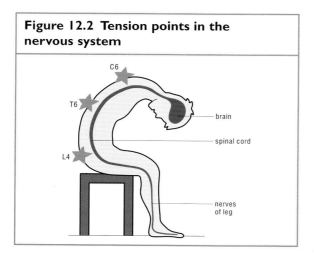

Figure 12.2 Tension points in the nervous system

C6

T6

L4

brain

spinal cord

nerves of leg

The nervous system, however, does not move consistently along its whole length as tension points occur (*see* fig 12.2). These are at the level of the sixth cervical vertebra, the sixth thoracic vertebra, and the fourth lumbar vertebra. With flexion, *tethering* (attachment) at these points means the spinal cord will be stretched towards the neck and lumbar spine, but away from the thoracic spine.

Parts of the nervous system can also move in relation to others, a process known as *intraneural movement.* For example, the spinal cord can slide within its containing sheath (dura mater), one nerve fibre within a bundle can move in relation to another, or an individual fibre can move in relation to its own sheath. In lateral flexion of the spine, the convex side of the spinal cord stretches in relation to the other, the difference in length being as much as 15 per cent.

In the case of gross movement, an injury that causes bruising or swelling over a region of the body may cause the nerve passing through this region to become adhered to other tissues. These types of injuries can range from bruising from a simple muscle pull affecting a nerve as it passes through the muscle, for example the sciatic nerve in relation to the hamstrings, to calluses from a healing

bone growing around the nerve, as in the case of the ulna nerve travelling around the outside of the elbow. These types of tethering will lead to nerve irritation and/or pain whenever the region is placed on stretch until the nerve breaks free. Intraneural movement may be limited if a crush injury causes swelling and scarring to regions of the nerve itself. If the individual nerve fibres within a bundle can no longer slide in relation to each other as a nerve is stretched around a corner, for example when bending the knee, tension and pain may result.

> **Key point** : Following any injury that causes bruising and swelling, nerves may be stuck down Anatomical tunnels (tethered) by clotted fluid.

Vulnerable areas of the nervous system

Nerves have several vulnerable areas (*see* fig 12.3).

Anatomical tunnels

These are tunnels formed through or around bone or soft tissues that have relatively rigid walls and are therefore unyielding. Excessive movement may cause a build-up of friction, especially in the presence of swelling within the tunnel from a minor injury. An example of a nerve tunnel is the median nerve travelling through the tunnel made by the small wrist (carpal) bones. This area, called the *carpel tunnel*, can give rise to 'carpal tunnel syndrome', a condition in which pressure on the medial nerve as it travels into the wrist gives aching and tingling sensations in the hand.

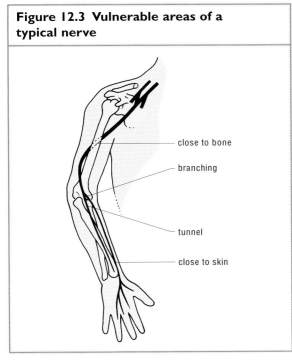

Figure 12.3 Vulnerable areas of a typical nerve

- close to bone
- branching
- tunnel
- close to skin

Nerve branches

A nerve is at risk when it branches, especially when this branching construction forms an acute angle. An example of this configuration is the digital nerve branching into the fourth and fifth toes. Pressure on this area through incorrect footwear can cause tissue tension and the development of a small cyst called a *digital neuroma*. This painful condition gives a burning sensation in the fourth and fifth toes due to nerve pressure.

Fixation points

The fixation points of the nervous system will not allow the normal sliding of nerves against underlying tissues and pressure near these points will be poorly tolerated. An example of a fixation point is at the head of the fibula bone where the common peroneal nerve wraps itself

around it. Damage to this area is common, for example from a direct blow from a football boot or hockey ball. The resultant swelling and scarring tethers the nerve, giving symptoms of injury.

Friction points

At certain points the nerves pass over or close to unyielding structures. Any tension will cause the nerve to give, but this will be limited. An example is where the brachial nerves extend from the cervical spine and pass over the first rib before travelling into the arm. Carrying heavy shopping bags can pull the nerves down on to the rib, giving pain and tingling in the whole arm (brachial neuralgia).

Tension points

The classic tension points of the nervous system (*see* fig 12.2) will cause the movement direction of the nerves to change, and are potential areas of concern. The sixth thoracic vertebra and the posterior aspect of the knee are examples, and these points are frequently a source of neural pain when stretching (*see* table 12.1).

Effects of stretching the nervous system

Stretching a nerve has many effects: some that aid healing, and some that can be damaging.

Healing effects

After an injury that causes swelling, a nerve stretch will move the nerve past the swollen area preventing the clotted swelling from sticking (adhering) to the nerve. In addition, any swelling within the nerve between its individual

Table 12.1	Vulnerable areas of the nervous system
Anatomical tunnels	A tunnel has relatively rigid, unyielding walls and, therefore, the nerve is susceptible to pressure, e.g. median nerve traveling through the wrist (carpel tunnel)
Nerve branches	When a nerve branches at an acute angle its gliding mechanism is reduced. There is, therefore, less movement available to it, e.g. digital nerve branching into the fourth and fifth toes.
Fixation points	Fixation points are less yielding and nerves are more likely to be injured by tension at these points, e.g. common peroneal nerve wrapping around the head of the fibula.
Friction points	Where a nerve passes close to unyielding tissues, there is an increased likelihood of pressure, e.g. brachial plexus nerves passing over the first rib.
Tension points	Points where the direction of neural movement is reversed, e.g. sixth thoracic vertebra and posterior aspect of the knee.

fibres may also be dispersed by pressure changes brought about through rhythmic stretching. Following chronic injury, a nerve may become tethered to underlying structures: stretching can break the nerve free of its binding scar tissue and allow nerve impulses to pass unimpeded once more. Rhythmic movement will also improve the blood supply to the nerve, and with it the amount of oxygen reaching the nervous tissue. In addition, the transport system within the nerve, called *axonal transport*, will be improved by movement and reduced by prolonged inactivity.

Damaging effects

Repeated stretching

As with muscle and bone, the physical stresses involved with repeated stretching will cause minor injury (microtrauma), which will encourage the tissue to adapt and become stronger. However, caution is necessary with repeated microtrauma: if the degree of physical stress exceeds the capacity of the nerve (or any tissue) to adapt, tissue breakdown and injury may result.

Continuous stretching

When a nerve is stretched continuously, for example by poor posture, its blood flow may be impaired. As the stretch is placed on, the blood vessels supplying the nerve become thinner. With just 8 per cent lengthening of the nerve, blood flow to the nerve begins to reduce substantially, and when the nerve is stretched by 15 per cent, the blood flow is completely cut off. If this happens only once, or if the nerve is released, allowed to recover, and then stretched again, no problem will arise.

However, prolonged blood flow reduction can cause problems. Initially, the reduction in blood flow causes the blood within the vessels to stagnate, and all the oxygen within it is rapidly used up. This oxygen starvation is known as *hypoxia*, and the result is often pain and pins and needles that reduces when the blood flow is reinstated. Crossing the legs for prolonged periods in the cinema is a good example of neural hypoxia. When the legs are released, a shower of pins and needles ensues, followed by warmth and a return of normal sensation when full oxygen levels are rebuilt. If the hypoxia remains, however, permanent injury may result: the lining of the small blood capillaries can become damaged and proteins can leak out into the surrounding area, causing a change in fluid pressure leading to local swelling, which being unable to escape, spreads along the length of the nerve. The swelling may eventually clot, causing a build-up of scar tissue within the area. The scarring will often stick to surrounding structures, preventing the nerve from sliding properly with everyday movements and causing friction as the nerve passes through tunnels and across other structures. More damage and nerve irritation occurs and pain is the inevitable result. In this way, minimal damage is exacerbated and a minor problem in one area spreads, causing symptoms in other body-parts.

> **Key point:** Poor posture can place continuous stress on a nerve, reducing its blood supply and starving it of oxygen.

Prolonged stretching

Stretching over a prolonged period may actually cause the nerve to lengthen. Hamstring stretching, for example, may cause the sciatic nerve to lengthen permanently.

How to stretch the nerves

A number of positions will cause tension build-up in the nervous tissue. Sometimes these positions are similar to classic stretches, and on other occasions they add subtle changes to a movement to apply a further stretch. In all cases, it must be remembered that nerves are delicate structures that must be treated with respect. Any nerve stretch may cause not just a feeling of tightness and aching, but pins and needles as well. This indicates that a stretch is working, but is too harsh. If this occurs, the stretch should be released slightly so that the feeling is just short of producing pins and needles. Over time, as the nerve stretches further, the point at which pins and needles occurs will move further away as the range of motion possible is increased.

Most of the stretches detailed below are combinations of several movements. When a nerve is adhered and causing problems, the stretch should begin with the distal movement, away from the tight structures. For example, if a combination of trunk flexion, straightening the leg and pulling the foot up (*see* the Classic Slump, exercise 127 below) causes problems in someone who is recovering from low back pain, the stretch should be released by allowing the knee to bend and the back to straighten slightly. Further stretch is gradually added by first pulling the foot up into dorsiflexion and then straightening the knee. Only at the last moment should the hip be flexed or the trunk bent further. After stretching, nervous tissue will need to recover in the same way that a muscle does. Remember that stretching a nerve reduces its blood flow, so adequate recovery must be allowed for. For this reason, nerve stretches should only be practised on alternate days, and a gentle warmth and general feeling of stretch is all that is required. Nerve stretches that cause pain are too extreme.

> **Key point:** When stretching a nerve, the movement must be gentle. Stretch just short of the point where you feel tingling (pins and needles). As soon as you feel this, release the stretch slightly and hold the position for up to 30 seconds.

Exercise 127   The Classic slump

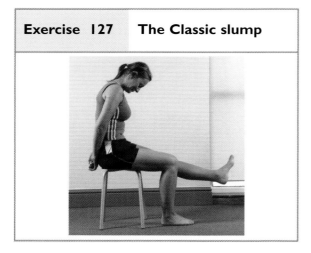

Starting position and instructions

Sit on a stool and link your arms behind your back. Gently flex your spine, beginning with your neck. At the same time straighten one of your legs, moving your foot up and your leg into a horizontal position.

Variations

Components of this action may be used individually at first, then built up into a full sequence. If one leg is very tight, keep that knee bent and gradually work towards straightening it, easing into the tightness but not forcing the movement. This can be achieved by placing the tight leg on top of the other and using the lower leg to provide a passive stretch while the upper leg relaxes. Alternatively, support the foot of the tight leg on the floor by placing it on a shiny piece of paper. With the weight of the leg taken through the floor, slide the foot forwards and backwards, again gradually working towards the fully extended position.

Points to note

This action stretches the whole of the nervous system, affecting the spinal cord, upper limb nerves and lower limb nerves of the straightened leg. As soon as you feel any tingling or resistance to the stretch, release the movement by flexing the leg slightly. Maintain this position for 20–30 seconds and then release. For the next repetition, again go just short of the point of pain/tingling hoping to push this point further away enabling you to straighten your leg further.

Exercise 128   Unsupported slump

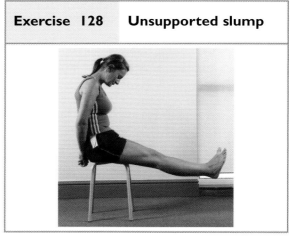

Starting position and instructions

Sit on the edge of a table with your feet together and unsupported. Link your hands behind you and gently flex your spine, beginning with your neck, to take your chin down to your chest. Continue the movement, rolling through the spine rather than leaning forwards. At the same time, straighten both legs, locking your knees and pulling your feet towards you. Maintain the full stretch for 30 seconds, then slowly release.

Variations

Components of this movement can be used individually at first and built up into the full sequence. Begin by flexing your trunk and linking your hands behind you. Next, remain upright initially and straighten both knees, pulling your feet towards you. Once both movements can be performed with no pain/tingling, combine the two into a single action.

Points to note

This action stretches the whole of the nervous system, affecting the spinal cord, upper limb nerves and lower limb nerves of both legs. As soon as you feel any tingling or resistance to the stretch, release the movement by flexing your legs slightly and releasing the neck flexion. Maintain this new position for 20–30 seconds and then release. For the next repetition, again go just short of the point of pain/tingling, hoping to push this point further away enabling you to straighten your legs further while maintaining your trunk flexion.

Exercise 129	Slump – long sitting

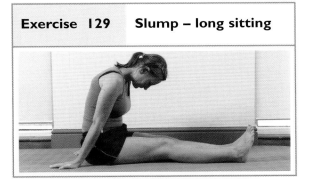

Starting position and instructions

The exercise is best performed close to a wall, with the feet pressed against the wall to dorsiflex them. Keeping your legs locked out straight, place your hands beside your knees and gradually flex your spine, beginning with the chin to the chest and rolling through the spine, aiming your head towards your hips rather than your knees.

Variations

You can use a yoga belt placed below the balls of your feet instead of the wall. Grip the belt and pull lightly, encouraging your trunk into thoracic flexion and your feet into dorsiflexion.

Points to note

Normally, good exercise practice would dictate that spinal alignment be maintained and excessive thoracic flexion avoided. However, the long sitting slump is designed to increase the emphasis on the thoracic spine, and so *controlled* thoracic flexion is actively encouraged in this movement.

Exercise 130	Rollover

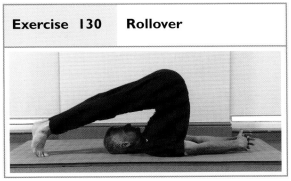

Starting position and instructions

The rollover is the classic yoga position called the Plough (*Halasana*). Lie on the floor on your back and bring your bent legs up over your head, leaving your arms on the floor. Pull your feet towards you (dorsiflexion) and gradually straighten your legs, trying to place your toes on the floor to take some of your body-weight.

Variations

If you are unable to place your toes on the floor, rest your feet on one or two cushions. With your arms wide, the surface area of support (footprint) is greater. Gripping the hands together reduces the surface area of support, but increases the effect of the stretch to the arms.

Points to note

The rollover has a similar effect to the long sitting slump, but places greater pressure on the thoracic spine and further forces the stretch. This is a specialised neural stretch that is contraindicated in a general exercise programme. If you have a history of lower back pain, you should only attempt it after consulting a physiotherapist.

Exercise 131	Straight leg raise – neural emphasis

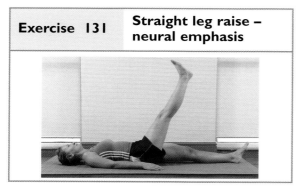

Starting position and instructions

Lie on the floor on your back and flex one hip, slowly raising the straight leg. At the same time, pull your toes towards you (dorsiflexion). Maintain the full stretch position for 20–30 seconds, then slowly lower.

Variations

The neural component of this stretch is increased by dorsiflexing the foot further, adducting the straight leg and flexing the neck to 'wind up' the spinal cord from above.

Points to note

The straight leg raising (SLR) movement is used as a test when a person has back pain. The aim is to see if the action produces pain from the back into the buttock and down the leg into the foot. If this is the case, it follows that the sciatic nerve is trapped; this is caused frequently by an inter-vertebral disc that has bulged or burst into the path of the nerve root at its junction with the spinal cord. The SLR action is a good illustration of the various stages of nerve movement that occur as a stretching exercise is performed. As the leg is raised initially, the sciatic nerve slides through a notch in the pelvis; as the leg is raised further, between 20–30 degrees of hip flexion, the nerve roots start to move past the individual vertebrae. Movement of the nerve past neighbouring structures stops altogether as the leg is raised past 70 degrees.

Figure 12.4 Effects of straight leg raising (SLR): (a) movement of sciatic nerve begins at the pelvis; (b) movement of roots begins at the spine; (c) minimal movement only, but increase in tension

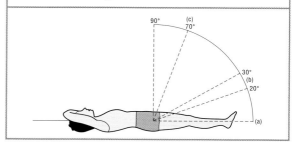

From this position to the full range stretch of 90 degrees, the nerve is stretched like an elastic band. Sliding of the nerve, therefore, occurs below 70 degrees, with stretching only coming on from this range to the end of the straight leg raise movement (*see* fig 12.4).

The SLR action is useful for mobilising and then stretching the sciatic nerve when its normal free motion is reduced, frequently as a result of previous back pain.

Exercise 132	Active knee extension – neural emphasis

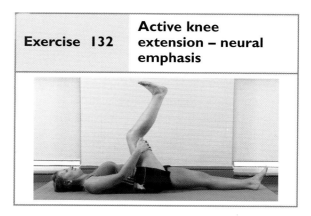

Starting position and instructions

Lie on the floor on your back, flex one of your hips and knees and place your hands behind your knee. Straighten your leg, keeping your knee directly above your hip.

Variations

Greater stress is placed on the nerve, rather than the hamstring muscles, by medially rotating your hip and pulling your foot towards your body (dorsiflexion).

Points to note

Make sure that your knee stays directly above your hip. There is a tendency with this movement to allow your knee to drop downwards so that your leg can be locked. However, the downward movement of the knee actually releases the stretch by reducing hip flexion.

Exercise 133	Straight leg raise – using doorway – neural emphasis

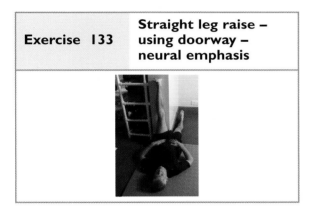

Starting position and instructions

Lie in a doorway with one leg straight along the floor and the other positioned with the heels on the doorframe. Gradually straighten the wall-supported leg by sliding your heel upwards, keeping it in contact with the doorframe. At the same time, dorsiflex your foot and place overpressure from the hand on to the knee to encourage the last few degrees of movement. The full stretch should be held for 30 seconds.

Variations

As a progression, both legs can be stretched at once by placing them both on the wall.

Points to note

If your heel is allowed to leave the wall support, the stress placed on your spine can be considerable as the low back may be forced into an extension equivalent to a bilateral straight leg raise. At all times, keep your heel in contact with the doorframe or wall.

Exercise 134	Femoral nerve stretch

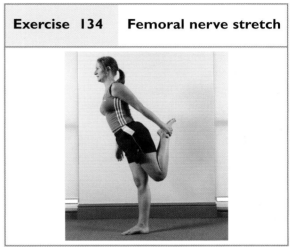

Starting position and instructions

Standing, flex one of your knees and pull your hip back into extension. At the same time, flex your trunk (spine) and bring your chin down on to your chest (cervical flexion).

Variations

This movement can also be performed lying on your side, in which case the upper leg is the one that is stretched.

Points to note

This is a variation of the rectus femoris stretch (*see* exercise 7). In that stretch, the trunk is kept upright to emphasise the effect on the muscle. In the femoral nerve stretch however, the nerve is emphasised by flexing the trunk and cervical spine.

| Exercise 135 | Brachial nerve stretch | Exercise 136 | Radial nerve stretch |

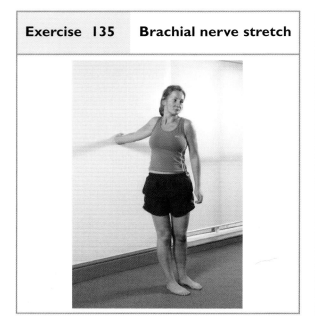 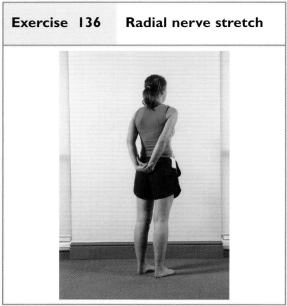

Starting position and instructions

Stand side on to a wall and place your hand on the wall at shoulder height, with your fingers horizontal and facing backwards. Slowly turn your body and head away from the wall, straightening your arm as you do so.

Variations

Pressing down on the stretched shoulder (depression) with the other hand will increase the stretch further.

Points to note

In the arm, three nerves need to be stretched: the radial nerve, the medial nerve and the ulnar nerve. Since all three come from the spinal cord in the thoracic region, they form a meshwork of nerve roots called the *brachial plexus*. The nerves of the brachial plexus are often stretched by a physiotherapist using the upper limb tension test (ULTT) in the same way that the SLR is used to stretch the lower limb nerves.

Starting position and instructions

Begin standing and keeping your shoulder down, adduct your right arm, rotating it inwards to place it behind the small of your back. Flex your wrist and pronate your forearm. Take hold of your wrist with your other hand and press your wrist into further flexion.

Variations

The stretch can be increased by flexing your neck (looking downwards). Shrugging your shoulders (scapular elevation) reduces the stretch.

Points to note

This exercise stretches the wrist extensors on the back of the forearm. To increase the emphasis on the nerve itself, the cervical flexion is important.

Exercise 137	Median nerve stretch

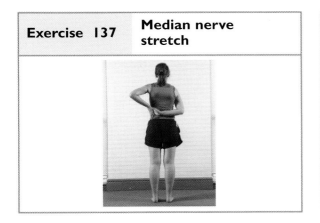

Exercise 138	Ulnar nerve stretch

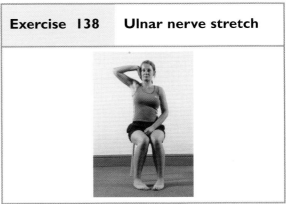

Starting position and instructions

Begin standing and, keeping your shoulder down, adduct your right arm and rotate it outwards. Extend your wrist and supinate your forearm. Take hold of your wrist with your other hand and press your wrist into further extension.

Variations

The stretch can be increased by flexing your neck (looking downwards). Shrugging your shoulders (scapular elevation) reduces the stretch.

Points to note

This exercise stretches the wrist flexors on the front of the forearm. To increase the emphasis on the nerve itself, the cervical flexion is important.

Starting position and instructions

Begin sitting and, keeping your shoulder down, abduct your right arm and flex it at the elbow to reach your hand to the side of your head, as though placing the flat of your hand over your ear.

Variations

The stretch can be increased by flexing your neck sideways away from your stretched arm.

Points to note

If the ulnar nerve is very tight, pins and needles will be felt on the outside of the elbow over the 'funny bone'.

Summary

- There are two types of nerve cell: those that carry electrical impulses and those that protect and support the nerves.
- All the nerves and the spinal cord are linked into a 'continuous tissue tract'.
- Nerves will slide as a limb is stretched.
- After injury, sticky swelling will 'tether' a nerve, reducing its normal movement.
- A nerve has several vulnerable areas where it may be trapped or its movement restricted.
- When a nerve is stretched, its blood flow is reduced. Repeated nerve stretches should therefore be avoided.
- Nerve stretching exercises resemble muscle stretches, but with subtle changes. They must be exact.
- When stretching a nerve, hold the stretch position at a point just short of feeling tingling or pain.

STRETCHING THE FASCIA

13

The concept of working on fascia has a long history in the physical therapies. It was first discussed in the work of Ida Rolf in America, who described a type of bodywork she called 'structural integration'. Most recently, this work has been championed by Tom Myers, Leon Chaitow and Judith DeLany. Myers has produced an excellent book in which he maps the *myofascial meridians*, and has a number of videos dealing with this subject under the name 'Anatomy Chains'. Chaitow and DeLany have produced two in-depth text books dealing with fascial treatment, or 'neuromuscular technique' (NMT). Much of the information for this chapter is taken from these publications, and the reader is referred to them for a more detailed study of this subject. All are listed in the references at the end of the book.

What is fascia?

The body is composed of four basic types of tissue: epithelial, connective, muscular and nervous (*see* table 2.2, page 21). Epithelial tissue covers surfaces or forms structures; for example, it makes up the glands and digestive system. Connective tissue consists of disparate cells floating within an extracellular matrix; depending on the cells present, connective tissue may form cartilage, bone or fascia. Muscular tissue contracts; it forms the muscles we train in the gym, as well as the muscles of the heart and those controlling the hair follicles in the skin. Nervous tissue makes up our nerves, spinal cord and brain.

To find out more about fascia, we need to focus on the connective tissue. Connective tissue is made up of fat (storage) and fibrous tissue (structure). The fibrous tissue contains collagen (white), a strong tough substance that gives the tissue its strength, and elastin (yellow), which gives the tissue its spring. Depending on the concentration of collagen and elastin, the connective tissue is either tough or pliable. Tendons, ligaments and the membranes covering bones and certain portions of the fascia contain mainly white fibres, whereas specific fascia such as the ligamentum flavum in the neck and the wall of blood vessels are mainly yellow elastic tissue.

So, fascia is a type of connective tissue. It links parts of the body together and transmits some of the force created by the muscles. More importantly, it provides a continuous tract covering several bones and muscles leading to a 'line of pull' that is not restricted to a single muscle.

Types of fascia

Fascia itself is subdivided into two types, superficial and deep. The superficial fascia lies just beneath the skin, acting as a base to enable the skin to move freely over the underlying tissues. A loosely arranged, folded meshwork with the folds filled with fat, the superficial fascia dictates the body contours and gives each of us our unique look. This portion of the fascia is the main place where fat is deposited in obesity, hence the use of skin-fold measurements to assess body-fat percentage.

The fat within the superficial fascia provides us with insulation and is very important in preventing heat loss, especially as we are smooth skinned rather than furry like a cat. Interestingly, in most other mammals (i.e. those with fur), the superficial fascia does not contain fat. For this reason, the skin of a cat is only loosely connected to the underlying tissue, which is why you can pick the animal up by the scruff of its neck. This is not the case with a person; the skin is too tight! On its under-surface, the superficial fascia becomes more fibrous and forms a distinct layer, which normally then connects to the deep fascia.

The deep fascia is tougher and more fibrous than the superficial fascia and surrounds almost every structure in the body. The deep fascia tends to be laid down in the direction of stress and attaches itself to bony projections as it passes over them. The under-surface of the deep fascia travels between muscle layers as the *intermuscular septa*, separating the groups of muscles from each other. The muscles are thus grouped in 'compartments' (*see* fig 13.1). In the case of the arms, these are the flexor and extensor compartments, and in the thigh they are the flexor, extensor and adductor compartments, for example.

The fascial membrane takes on a variety of names depending on its anatomical position. Around the brain and spinal cord it is the *meninges*, around the heart it is the *pericardium*, within the abdomen it is called the *peritoneum* and around the bones, it is known as the *periosteal*. Even within the musculo-skeletal system fascia may be specialised. At the side of the leg we have the ilio-tibial band (ITB) and in the back the thoraco-lumbar fascia (TLF). The important feature, however, is that all of the layers of fascia are connected to each other. Fascia is really a 'soft tissue skeleton', as it supports the body, forms boundaries and moulds the shape of

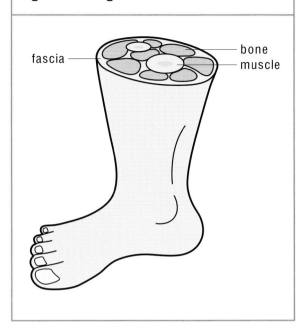

Figure 13.1 A gross muscle fascia

fascia — bone
muscle

the body tissues. It is not really possible to perform a stretching exercise and affect only one muscle; when we stretch, one muscle may receive the greater stretching effect, but both the muscle and the fascia will change tension. For this reason, we can talk of muscle and fascia as a single inseparable unit called *myofascia*.

Key point: Fascia is our 'soft tissue skeleton', posterior surface forming a continuous covering that links our bones, joints and muscles together.

Fascial pathways

According to Myers (2001), there are four main fascial pathways (*see* table 13.1). The superficial back line (SBL) supports the body in full extension, preventing it from collapsing into flexion. It is therefore important in forward bending and lifting tasks. The superficial front line (SFL) transmits muscle force to create powerful flexion of the legs and trunk. The lateral line (LL) is important for single leg actions during walking and running, as well as for lateral bending activities of the trunk. Finally, the spiral line (SL) creates rotational movements of the body, which are important during functional activities such as walking and running as well as during sport.

Each of the four major fascial pathways links a variety of myofascial structures, which are detailed in table 13.2. When performing any stretch, we can increase the emphasis on the fascial pathways by involving more of these structures. For example, when performing a sit-and-reach stretch (exercises 24 and 108), the stretch works the hamstrings and spine. The myofascial

Table 13.1	Fascial pathways
Pathway	Position
Superficial back line	Connects posterior surface of body from toes to knees and then knees to brow.
Superficial front line	Anterior body surface from top of feet to the sides of the skull.
Lateral line	Foot and outside of ankle along the lateral aspect of the leg and trunk to the ear.
Spiral line (*takes portions from other three*)	From one side of the skull, across the back to the opposite shoulder and then back across the chest and down the side of the body. From the foot up the back to rejoin the skull fascia.

Table 13.2	Fascial pathways in detail
Superficial back line	• Scalp • Erector spinae and thoroco lumbar fascia • Sacrotuberous ligament • Hamstrings • Gastrocnemius and Achilles • Plantarfascia and short toe extensors
Superficial front line	• Scalp • Sternomastoid • Sternal fascia • Rectus abdominis • Rectus femoris and quadriceps • Patellar tendon • Toe and foot extensors
Lateral line	• Sternomastoid and deep neck muscles • Intercostals • Lateral abdominals • Gluteus maximus • Tensor fascia lata • Hip abductors • Fibular ligament • Peroneal muscles
Spiral line	• Deep neck muscles (splenius) • Rhomboids • Serratus anterior • Oblique abdominals • Abdominal fascia • Ilio tibial tract (ITB) • Tibialis anterior • Peroneal longus • Biceps femoris • Sacrotuberous ligament • Erector spinae and thoroco-lumbar fascia

effect on the superficial back line can be increased by bending the spine, touching the chin to the chest and drawing the foot into dorsiflexion.

The superficial back line (SBL)

Exercise 139	Forward bend with belt

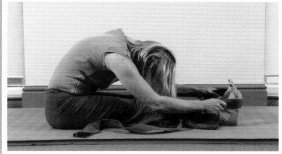

Starting position and instructions

Sit on a mat with your legs straight. Bend forwards from the waist, flexing the whole of your trunk and neck, and try to touch your chin to the top of your breastbone. At the same time, pull your feet and toes towards you (dorsiflexion of the ankle and extension of the toes).

Variations

To increase the intensity of the stretch, place a yoga belt or hand towel around your feet and toes and gently pull the toes towards you.

Points to note

This stretch targets the whole of the SBL, involving the plantarfascia, calf and hamstrings, then right up through the spine to the scalp. However, with over-pressure from the yoga belt or hand towel, the pressure within the lumbar discs will be increased. This is not recommended for individuals with a history of a disc lesion (slipped disc), unless supervised by a physiotherapist.

Exercise 140	Downward dog

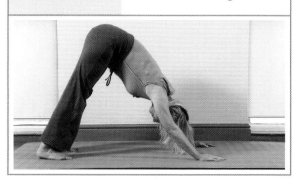

Starting position and instructions

Stand with your feet hip-width apart. Keeping your back straight, bend your knees and reach down to touch the floor with your flat hands. Keeping the hands in place, walk your feet backwards until they are 1–1½ m away from your hands and your body forms an upside down 'V'. Keep your arms straight and press your chest downwards to straighten your back.

Variations

Taking your feet further backwards will bring your legs closer to the horizontal and increase the angle of dorsiflexion at the ankle, placing a greater stretch on the calf and achilles. Bringing the feet closer to the head will releases some of the stretch on the calf and enable you to press your chest further down, increasing the stretch on the chest and shoulders.

Points to note

This is a classic yoga posture that stretches the SBL while taking some of the flexion stress away from the spine. If you find your feet slipping, practise the position with your heels against a wall. If you are unable to reach the floor, place your hands on a low bench (step bench) instead.

Superficial front line (SFL)

Exercise 141	Passive full spine extension with knee flexion

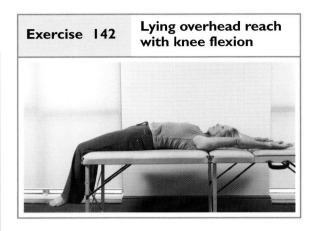

Exercise 142	Lying overhead reach with knee flexion

Starting position and instructions

Lie on a mat with your hands beneath your shoulders. Press down with your hands and straighten your arms, arching your back. When you get to the top of the movement, look up towards the ceiling (cervical extension) and bend your knees (knee flexion).

Variations

If you are unable to straighten your arms, place your arms further forwards (a forearm's length in front of the shoulder line) and slightly wider apart (1½ times wider than your shoulders).

Points to note

This exercise, like exercise 40, forces the lower back (lumbar region) into extension. Encouraging extension in the lumbar region is usually a good thing, unless you have a hollow back (lordotic posture). If this is the case, this movement may be painful, so stop if you feel pain rather than simply tightness in the lower back and seek advice from a physiotherapist or qualified personal trainer.

Starting position and instructions

Lie on a gym bench or bed with your bottom supported but your lower thighs off the bed. Bend your knees and at the same time reach overhead, trying to touch the bench above you.

Variations

The SFL stretch can be increased by placing the shoulders on a cushion so that the neck can lower into extension. In addition, pointing the toes and feet (plantarflexion and toe flexion) will target the toe and foot extensors, which form the lower part of the SFL.

Points to note

If you find it too difficult to stretch your arms overhead to touch the bench, place a pillow on the bench above your head and lower your arms onto that instead.

Lateral line (LL)

| Exercise 143 | **Supported side flexion with hip adduction** |

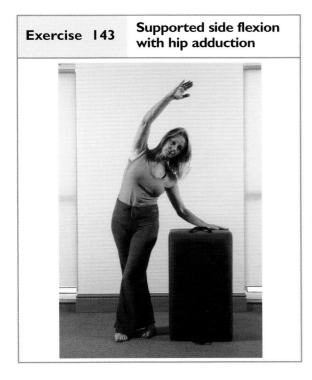

Starting position and instructions

Stand left side on to a table or high gym bench and place your left hand on the bench for support. Draw your right leg across and behind your left leg (hip adduction) and reach your right hand overhead, towards your right ear. Bend to the left, taking your body-weight through your left hand onto the tabletop, and move your left ear towards your left shoulder. Reverse the movement by bending to the right.

Variations

Although the complete movement stretches the whole of the LL, you can add the components gradually. First, perform the hip adduction with trunk side flexion. Second, perform the overhead reach and neck side flexion. When you are comfortable with both movements, combine the two into a single action as described above.

Points to note

It is common to have an asymmetrical body, so do not be surprised if one side of your body is stiffer than the other. Work on the stiffer side, aiming to regain symmetry rather than simply to increase the range of motion.

| Exercise 144 | **Side lying side flexion** |

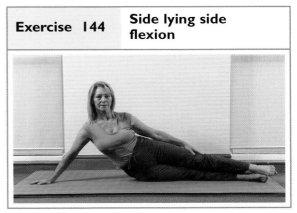

Starting position and instructions

Lie on your right side with a pad or folded towel beneath your lower hip (greater trochanter). Place your right hand beneath your right shoulder and press down, stretching your spine into lateral flexion. At the same time, reach your left arm along the outside of your left leg. When your trunk is upright, flex your neck to the left and take a deep breath to expand your ribcage.

Variations

If you are unable to lock your arm out straight, move it further away from your body.

Points to note

As with all side stretches, it is common to find that one side of your body is stiffer than the other. Work on the stiffer side, aiming to regain symmetry rather than increase the range of motion.

Spiral line

Exercise 145	Lying spinal rotation with leg straightening

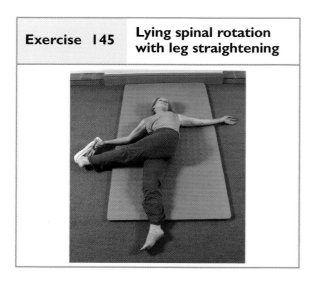

Exercise 146	Prone lying leg adduction with lateral flexion and rotation

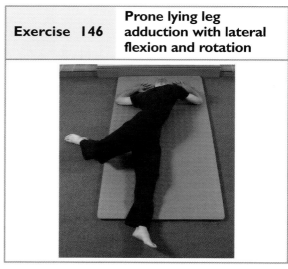

Starting position and instructions

Lie on the floor with your right leg bent and left leg straight. Tuck your left hip beneath you and twist your spine to the left, lowering your right knee to the floor. Gradually straighten your right leg and take hold of your shin or foot with your left hand. Keep your right arm on the ground straight out to the side and look to the right. Reverse the movement to target the left side.

Variations

If you find it difficult to hold your shin or foot, wrap a yoga belt or small towel around your shin and hold that instead.

Points to note

As you perform this exercise you will often note a 'click' or 'pop' from the spine. This is normally the release of gas bubbles within the small facet joints of the spine and is harmless. If the click is painful, however, stop the exercise and rest. If the pain continues, consult a physiotherapist.

Starting position and instructions '

Lie on your front with your arms out to your sides, bent at the elbow. Your chest and head should be flat on the floor. Lift your right leg and take it across your left (adduction). As you do this, allow your trunk to flex to the left and rotate slightly, opening the right side of your ribcage. Reverse the movement to focus on the left side of the body.

Variations

This movement may be combined with spinal extension (*see* exercise 40) to stretch the abdominal fascia as well as the oblique abdominals. To do this, place the hands under the shoulders and press into the ground to extend the spine, then come up onto the elbows or flat hands.

Points to note

If you have limited hip flexibility this movement may not be suitable. Where the hip does not extend easily, the lumbar spine tends to extend too much instead (hyperextension).

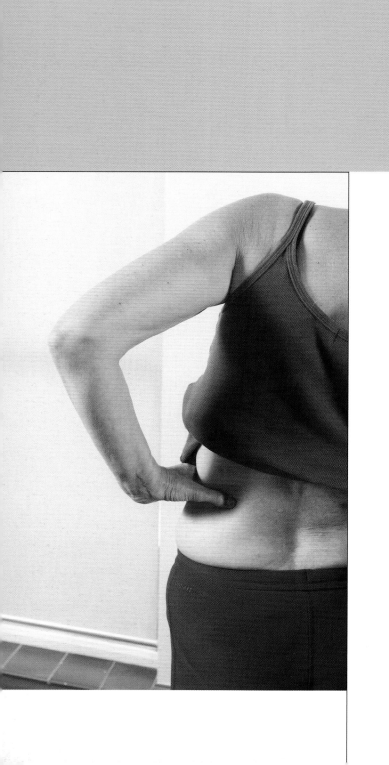

PART **THREE**

PRACTICAL
APPLICATION

3

TRIGGER POINTS

14

Trigger points (TrP) are highly sensitive focal areas within a tight muscle. They are often painful at rest, and can refer pain through an area, causing it to spread away from the TrP along a limb, for example. Take a TrP in the supraspinatus muscle at the top of the shoulder blade. This may be painful if someone digs their fingers into the area, and the pain may spread out across the upper back and even down into the arm. In severe cases, where the TrP is very active, pain may travel down the arm right into the fingers.

A TrP can be one of two types. One which is painful nearly all the time, and the client is aware of is called an *active* TrP. Sometimes, however, a client may have pain in an area which has been referred from a TrP which they were not aware of. In this case the TrP is said to be *latent*. In the case of the supraspinatus example above, the client may have been aware of arm pain but not the TrP at the top of the shoulder blade. In this case the supraspinatus TrP is latent.

> **Key point**: An active trigger point is one which a client is aware of. A latent TrP is one where the client is aware of general pain in another body area, made worse by pressing the TrP.

Trigger point development

A number of factors can lead to the development of a TrP (table 14).

Psychological factors typically include anxiety and stress, and lead to TrP development in the so-called 'emotional muscles'. These include the neck and shoulders, and lower back. Prolonged stress may lead to TrP development especially in the upper trapezius, and erector spinae. Biomechanical factors include posture. Sitting at a computer, slouched forwards, allows the scapulae to move outwards (scapular abduction) over stretching the rhomboid muscles.

Table 14	Important factors in trigger point development	
Psychosocial	**Biomechanical**	**Chemical**
Depression	Posture	Toxic chemicals
Anxiety	Trauma (sudden injury)	Nutrient deficiency
Stress	Overuse (gradual injury)	Allergic reaction
Fear		

This gives rise to rhomboid TrPs with local pain along the inner edge of the scapula. Muscle injury as a result of overuse or trauma can lead to TrP development, often giving secondary pain once the original injury has resolved. An example here would be a simple sprained ankle which damages the lateral ligament on the outside of the ankle. Initially pain and swelling occur at the ankle, but the peronei muscles along the outside of the shin will work hard to protect the ankle. The result can be a peroneus TrP some months after the original injury has resolved. Pain gives 'lateral shin splints' creating tightness over the outer shin after prolonged walking or running.

Interestingly, there are several biochemical factors which have been linked to TrP development. These include reactions to allergens and deficiencies in certain vitamins, especially the B vitamins. It is likely that these factors while not actually causing individual TrPs could make a person more susceptible to them. If a client is developing TrPs repeatedly in different muscles they should seek advice from their GP.

Physiology

Trigger points commonly begin when one of the muscle membranes is damaged either by repeated movements (overuse) or a sudden mistimed pull (trauma). The membrane damage alters the release of the chemical *acetycholine* which is involved in muscle contraction. This chemical is a *neurotransmitter* (nerve impulse chemical) which spreads across the muscle causing contraction when a nerve impulse arrives from the brain and spinal cord. The change in acetycholine release causes a parallel alteration in calcium levels at the junction (synapse) between the end of the nerve and the muscle – the so called 'neuromuscular junction'. Muscle contraction occurs because of the chemical imbalance which exists, and this contraction simply continues even though no nervous impulses are being sent out. When a muscle contracts normally, nerve impulses travel to the muscle and the resulting electrical impulses can be measured on an EMG machine. The stronger the contraction, the greater the signal (amplitude) of the EMG, but where a TrP exists, electrical activity is detected in the muscle even when no nervous impulses are present. This feature, called *spontaneous electrical activity* (SEA) is a measure which can be used in hospitals to identify a TrP and know when it has been successfully treated.

> **Key point**: Both chemical and electrical changes occur in a muscle which develops a trigger point.

The permanent contraction of a few local muscle fibres gives a nodule which is often felt when pressing into a TrP. The contraction restricts local blood flow allowing poisons to accumulate in the area giving a burning pain, typical of TrPs.

Because the nodule causes local contraction of a few muscle fibres, the bunching pulls on the muscle causing the second feature often seen with TrPs, a *taut band*. This appears like a cord within the muscle which you can flick your fingers over, and is a familiar feature to massage therapists.

> **Key point**: The two key features of a trigger point are a *nodule* within the muscle and a *taut band*.

Although TrPs are obviously painful, that is not their only feature. The chemical and mechanical changes which occur also cause the muscle to weaken, allowing further posture changes. Getting rid of the TrP is therefore a primary aim, in the short term it will relieve pain, but in the long term by allowing postural correction it can prevent further problems.

Identifying a trigger point

If you have a TrP yourself, you can usually feel it by pressing your fingers into the painful area. But, how can you identify a TrP in a client? Well, the tightening of the TrP restricts impulses conducted through local nerves. A nerve has a feeling (sensory) function giving pain, and a movement (motor) function giving muscle-weakness. However, the third characteristic of the nerve comes from its sympathetic nerve fibres. These control a number of features including skin condition. As a result subtle skin changes can be seen in the region of a long lasting TrP, especially on the back. These include altered regions of sweating making the skin tacky or powdery and dry. Skin puckering known as 'orange peel skin' is often noticeable, and there may be a change in the stretchiness of the skin itself. These characteristic types of skin appearance are known as *trophic changes*. To be seen they require close inspection and may be more easily identified by gently gliding your fingers over the skin surface.

> **Key point:** Trophic skin changes which occur when a TrP has been present for a prolonged period include dry powdery skin, tacky skin, skin puckering, and loss of elasticity.

Release Techniques

There are a number of techniques which we can use to get rid of a TrP and allow the muscle to stretch normally. These are used before stretching, or as part of a gentle stretching action. Once the TrP is released, the muscle must be slowly stretched to its optimal level, comparing it to the unaffected side of the body.

Ischaemic compression

Ischaemic compression is a local massage technique which you can apply to yourself or your partner. Often termed myofascial release, this technique uses a sustained pressure over a TrP which gradually distorts the tissues. By holding the pressure on for 90–120 seconds, the tissues gradually become more fluid. This is a little like pressing hard onto a piece of putty or plasticine. As you press, you will gradually feel the hardness of the TrP ease off and pain will subside. What is happening here is a reversal of the process which follows the onset of a TrP. We saw that blood flow is reduced as a result of TrP formation. This in turn causes dehydration of the tissues stiffening them. The ischaemic compression technique causes water molecules to seep back into the area, and as the pressure is released, fresh blood floods into the region.

Press using the flat of your fingers or your hand, and slide your fingers into the tissues along the muscle length. Initially, use a gentle pressure across the surface of the skin like massage. As tension eases, increase the pressure as though you were trying to actually stretch the skin. Finally, maintain the pressure over the TrP and apply a gentle stretch to the underlying muscle.

Positional release

Positional release works not by stretching a tight muscle, but by taking stress off the tissues so that the muscle can 're-set' itself and allow the TrP to release. The thought here is that prolonged occurrence of a TrP causes the body to 'remember' pain and exaggerate it even when the original cause of the pain has long gone. Positional release works by affecting the pain nerves and the positional (proprioceptive) nerves connected to the tissue with the TrP.

Get your client to press on the TrP and feel how painful it is. They should then move the limb around, until they find a position which reduces the pain of the TrP – the so-called '*position of ease*'. This new, less painful position is held for 90–120 seconds and then the TrP is re-assessed. Because tight muscles often full joints out of alignment, there may also be TrPs in the muscles opposite to that which is painful, so search these out as well.

PNF stretching

We have covered PNF stretching on page 57. We know that it is a technique which reduces tone in a muscle and so is ideal as a follow up to TrP release. Once the TrP begins to ease, use PNF stretching to normalise the tone in the affected muscle, and then emphasise correct alignment in general movements.

Targeting affected muscles

Exercise 147	Upper upper trapezius

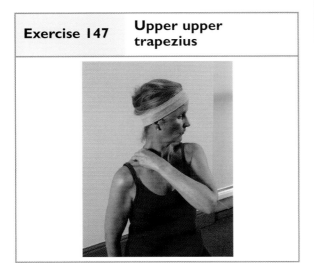

Starting position and instructions

Sit upright on a chair or gym bench. Rest your left hand over your right shoulder and tip your head to the left (left lateral flexion of the neck). Grip your three central fingers together into a single unit, and press this into the TrP within your trapezius muscle. Press the area gently while maintaining the stretched position. As the muscle pain subsides, increase the stretch by laterally flexing your neck further.

Variations

Flex or rotate your neck to vary the effect of the stretch. Actively depress the right shoulder blade (pull it downwards) to stabilise the scapula against the ribcage. Use a light massage stroke across the fibres of the muscle, from front to back.

Points to note

As you apply this stretch, make sure you do not flex the thoracic spine, or raise the right shoulder.

Exercise 148	Pec major

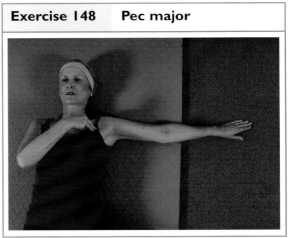

Starting position and instructions

Lie on your back on the floor. Move your left arm out to the side. Use your right hand to locate and press the trigger point within the muscle either close to the breastbone (the sternal head of pec major) or close to the collar bone (the clavicular head). Press the trigger point and stroke slowly along the muscle in a diagonal direction from chest to shoulder. As the trigger point releases allow the muscle to stretch further.

Variations

If your pec major is quite tight, rest your forearm on a cushion initially to reduce the stretch. As the muscle lengthens, stretch further to the floor. If, on the other hand, you are very flexible and find the floor stretch easy, lie on a gym bench and allow your arm to stretch below the horizontal level.

Points to note

When the pec major is tight you have a round shouldered posture. However, this normally goes with tightness of the upper (thoracic) spine as well, and this can be stretched using exercise 36.

Exercise 149	Pec minor

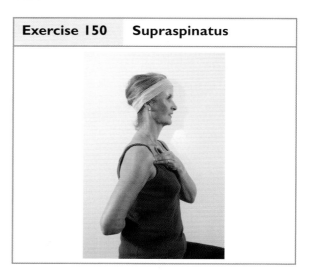

Starting position and instructions

Lie on the floor and get your training partner place a weight bag over the front of your shoulder so that your shoulder is pressed right

onto the floor. Find the ball of your shoulder joint with the fingers of your left hand and move your fingers downwards and inwards towards your feet until you hit the first couple of ribs. This is where you will find the pec minor trigger point. Press on it and maintain the pressure as you allow your shoulder to relax and be pressed further into the floor by the weight bag.

Variations

Lie on your front with your shoulder on a shallow cushion and allow your body weight to press your shoulder backwards.

Points to note

The pec minor muscle lifts your upper ribs when you take a very deep breath. To lengthen the muscle further, breath out forcefully as you apply the stretch.

Exercise 150	Supraspinatus

Starting position and instructions

Sit on a gym bench with your right hand behind the small of your back. Reach across your shoulder and place your fingers into the muscles at the top / back of your shoulder below the trapezius.

Gently press into this area until you find the trigger point and then massage it in a horizontal direction until it releases.

Variations

Use a contract-relax (CR) technique to release the muscle further. Press your forearm into your back (resisted lateral or outward rotation), hold this tension for 10–20 seconds and then release.

Points to note

The supraspinatus may develop two trigger points; one in its muscle belly at the top of the shoulder blade (scapula), the other at its insertion onto the top of the arm bone (humerus). To locate the humeral trigger point press on the front of the shoulder as you perform the stretch described above.

Exercise 151 Splenius capitus

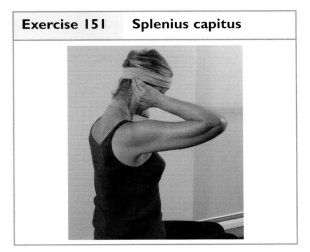

Starting position and instructions

Sit on a chair and place your fingertips on the area of your skull behind your ears. Gently draw your chin inwards as though trying to give yourself a double chin and try to look downwards at the top of your breastbone. By doing this you should lift the back of your head

upwards slightly in a rocking action (Pilates skull rock exercise). Gentle massage the tender trigger points in the muscle, and as they release pull the chin in further.

Variations

Where one muscle is tighter than the other, tip your head to that side (lateral flexion) and turn your head towards the muscle (rotation). The combination of lateral flexion and rotation with increase the stretch on the muscle.

Points to note

Splenius capitus is a small deep muscle which lies beneath the trapezius and sternomastoid. It travels from the lower neck to a bone behind your ear (mastoid process) and the lower rim of the back of your skull (nuchal line). Its importance lies in the fact that it develops tenderness and can be the cause of headaches if you spend a lot of time on a computer with your chin poked forwards.

Exercise 152 Rhomboids

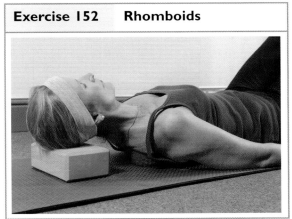

Starting position and instructions

Place a tennis ball on the floor and lie on your side so that the ball is level with the middle of your shoulder blades. Place the rhomboids on stretch by gripping your opposite shoulders, right hand to left shoulder and left to right. This 'self hugging' position will draw your shoulder blades apart (scapular abduction) and place the rhomboids on stretch. Roll from your side to your back so that the tennis ball is squashed beneath your back. Shuffle so that the ball is placed between your spine and the inner edge of your shoulder blade, over the most painful area which is the trigger point. Allow your bodyweight to press you downwards and maintain the position for 90–120 seconds breathing normally (make sure you don't hold your breath).

Variations

You may use a golf ball instead of a tennis ball. This will give a greater pressure as it is harder, but be careful not to rest your spinal bones on the ball.

Points to note

The rhomboid trigger point may form when the muscle is lengthened rather than shortened, in a round shouldered position. This is because the scapulae move apart, and the rhomboid muscles are trying hard to hold the scapulae back, but failing (eccentric muscle action). You are therefore trying to release the trigger point and reduce muscle pain with this exercise, rather than simply lengthen the muscle.

Exercise 153	Quadratus lumborum (QL)

Starting position and instructions

Stand side on to a high bench or table with your left side to the outside. Bend over sideways towards the table and support yourself on your right hand. Draw your left hand up and press your thumb into the muscles between your pelvis and lower ribs, midway between your spine (erector spinae) and the side of your body (obliques). Find the trigger point and compress it for 90–120 seconds. As your muscle releases and the trigger point pain reduces, allow yourself to sidebend further.

Variations

You may also perform this exercise side bent over a gym ball, using your upper hand to locate and release the trigger point.

Points to note

To fully stretch the QL, you must move your pelvis and ribcage apart. In standing this can be better achieved by dipping your hip on the tight side so that the pelvis tips down laterally to this side. When taking a deep breath, the QL pulls the lower rib downwards to help fill the lungs fully. To increase the stretch on the muscle, exhale fully to allow the lower rib to move up.

Exercise 154   Erector spinae

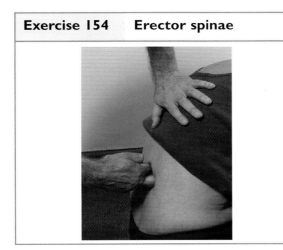

Exercise 155   Piriformis

Starting position and instructions

Sit on the floor with your knees bent to 90 degrees, your training partner kneeling behind you. Locate a painful trigger point within the bulk of the erector spinae to the side of the spine. Get your training partner to press into this area using their knuckle or elbow, as you bend (flex) your spine moving your head towards your upper thighs.

Variations

Your training partner may also stand behind you and place their knee into the trigger point. Combine flexing and rotation of your spine, moving your head towards your opposite thigh.

Points to note

When you stretch in this way there is a greater emphasis on the upper portion of the erector spinae. If your trigger point is very low down close to your pelvis, an alternative stretch is to lie on the floor and bring your knees into your chest, lifting your tailbone from the floor (posterior pelvic tilt).

Starting position and instructions

Lie on the floor and place a tennis ball beneath your right (painful) buttock. Move around until the ball presses into your painful trigger point. Compress the trigger point until the pain subsides, and then draw your leg up placing your right hand on your right knee and hold your right foot with your left hand. Impart the stretch onto piriformis by drawing your foot towards you and pressing your knee away. This action will rotate your hip joint outwards (lateral rotation) while keeping it in a bent (flexed) position.

Variations

Rather than using your hands, you can perform the stretch using the knee of your other leg. See gluteal stretch, exercise 2.

Points to note

This muscle lies over the sciatic nerve, the major nerve that passes through your buttock and into your thigh. It is common for compression of this area to give tingling (pins and needles) into your leg. If this occurs, release the pressure slightly until the tingling goes away.

Exercise 156   Hamstrings

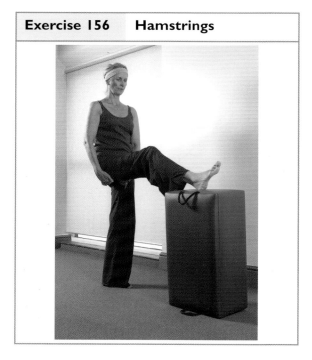

Starting position and instructions

Stand with your painful leg bent and heel resting on a low bench or table below waist height. Push your fingers into the trigger point on the back of your thigh, as the pain subsides, gently press your leg straighter by sliding your heel out along the bench.

Variations

A greater stretch is given using a higher bench, and sliding the leg slightly sideways outwards (hip abduction) or inwards (hip adduction) will change the emphasis of the stretch.

Points to note

The upper portion of the hamstrings will receive a greater stretch using an anterior tilt of the pelvis (tail forwards) rather than a posterior tilt (tipping your tail backwards).

Exercise 157   TFL/ITB

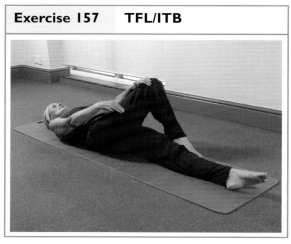

Starting position and instructions

Lie on your back and bend your painful (right leg). Bend your left leg and cross it over your right. Locate your painful trigger point on the side of your thigh and press it until the pain subsides. Stretch the TFL/ITB by using the weight of your top (left) leg to press your bottom (right) leg across your body into adduction.

Variations

Varying the bend at the knee will alter the emphasis of the stretch. The ITB/TFL may also be stretched using a partner stretch exercise 102.

Points to note

The stretch on the ITB/TFL must be maintained for a long period 2–3 minutes to get the full effect.

MEASURING FLEXIBILITY

15

Why we need to measure flexibility

Flexibility should be measured in order to:
• determine your existing range of motion;
• assess any muscle imbalance;
• chart your progress as you train.

Range of motion

When a muscle is more flexible than normal (hyperflexible), there is no need to stretch it, and in fact to do so could leave you open to injury. If a muscle is too flexible, there may not be enough strength in the muscles supporting the joint to control the total range of motion, in such a case, we say that *hyperflexibility* (greater than normal range of motion) has developed into *instability* (inability to control joint alignment through the whole available range).

> **Key point**: Hyperflexibility is simply a greater continue, although the muscles, in general, would amount of flexibility than the average person. Instability is the inability to control and maintain the detected, the answer is to stretch only those muscles alignment of a joint.

Muscle imbalance

You will also need to assess the ratio of muscle flexibility on one side of the joint to that on the opposing side. When there is a marked difference in flexibility or strength between the two, muscle imbalance is present (*see* page 00) and it would be wrong to practise an overall stretching programme. This would simply allow the imbalance to continue, although the muscles, in general, would all be more flexible. When an imbalance is detected, the answer is to stretch only those muscles that are too tight, and to strengthen and shorten those that are too loose (flabby) by exercising in the inner-range position. Once the imbalance has been corrected, a general flexibility programme can be used.

Charting progress

Stretching is a long-term part of any training programme, so you will need 'goals' or targets to aim for. In order to do this, you will need to *measure* your flexibility and aim at improving it within a certain *time*. For example, you might aim at improving the range of motion of a joint by a certain number of degrees in a certain number of months; or aim to reach far enough to touch a certain point by a set date (for instance, Christmas or birthdays). Either way, the goals you set yourself must be specific and realistic. It is no good simply saying that you want to increase your flexibility, because this is too open-ended: increase it by how much, and in how long? Your goals must also be realistic: you may never be able to perform the splits if you are over 50 and very inflexible in the hip adductors. This really does not matter, provided that your degree of flexibility is appropriate to your age, body make-up and activity level. Remember, the right amount of stretching is the right amount for you as an individual. There is no competition – no winners and no losers. When goals are set, you are only really competing with yourself, so the goals must be acceptable to you.

Key point: When setting goals, the mnemonic SMART is useful. Your goals should be Specific, Measurable, Acceptable, Realistic and Timed.

How to measure flexibility

Using a score chart

The score chart, illustrated in table 15.1, can be used as a test to measure your flexibility. Average values are quoted, but they are for general guidance only. If you have a specific problem that limits your flexibility, you should see your physiotherapist or personal trainer.

You should perform a warm-up before testing any movement, and wear warm clothing to keep your body warm while performing the tests. Make sure that you perform the same degree of warm-up each time you measure your flexibility. The exercises are either active or static stretches (see pages 57 and 58) and should be performed slowly and held in the stretched position. There should be no bobbing or bouncing actions, which will give a deceptively high score. The instructions for each exercise are included in the table.

Clinical flexibility testing

The score chart can only give a rough, but still very useful, guide to flexibility. Where a more precise measurement is needed, clinical testing

is used. This accurately measures the angle of the joint at the point of maximal stretch, and is called *goniometry*. A number of goniometers are available. The simplest is the *universal goniometer* (*see* fig 15.2). This consists of a 180-degree or 360-degree protractor. It has a single axis and scale, but two arms. One arm is held stationary, the axis of the goniometer is placed on the axis (centre) of the joint to be measured, and the two arms rest on the mid-lines of the bones on either side of the joint. The joint angle obtained when stretching is read from the centre scale.

The *gravity goniometer* consists of a needle inside a fluid-filled container. The needle points downwards due to gravity and acts as a reference against which the joint range is measured. The goniometer is strapped on to the limb and a direct reading is achieved.

If you want to measure your flexibility when-performing a certain sports action, the simplest way is to take a picture of the action and then to measure the movement on the photograph. This is made easier by drawing lines along the long axis of the bones and the using a simple school protractor to measure the angle between the two lines. Remember however, that the angle of the camera can change the appearance of the limbs and so to be truly objective you should really position the camera in the same position each time you take a photograph of a particular action.

How to use the goniometer

Figure 15.2 shows the plan for a simple goniometer. Photocopy this, stick the copy on to a piece of firm card or plastic and cut out the shape. Fasten the two pieces together with a clip. The goniometer is now ready for use.

To take a reading, position point A over the centre of rotation of the joint. This is the point of the joint around which the movement appears to take place. Figure 15.1 shows the

Figure 15.1 Joint centres

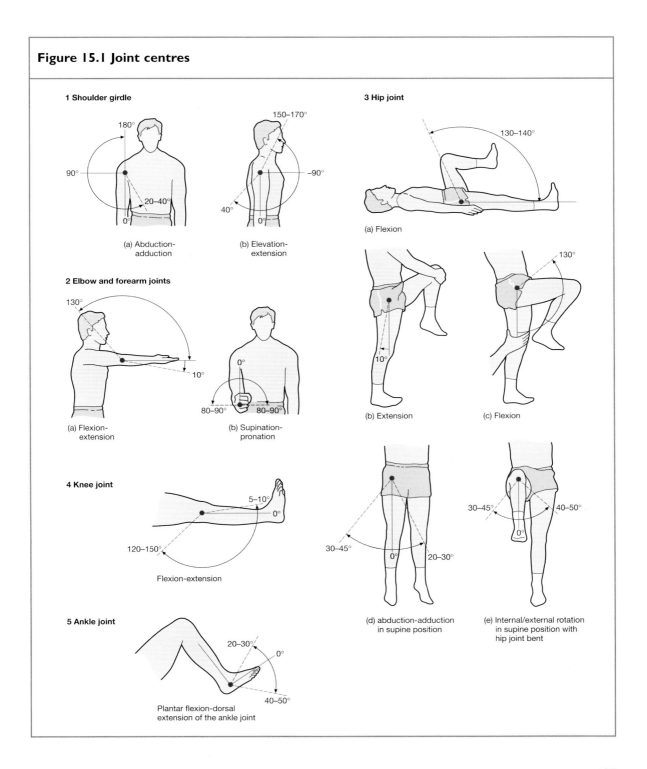

1 Shoulder girdle

(a) Abduction-adduction

(b) Elevation-extension

2 Elbow and forearm joints

(a) Flexion-extension

(b) Supination-pronation

3 Hip joint

(a) Flexion

(b) Extension

(c) Flexion

(d) abduction-adduction in supine position

(e) Internal/external rotation in supine position with hip joint bent

4 Knee joint

Flexion-extension

5 Ankle joint

Plantar flexion-dorsal extension of the ankle joint

Figure 15.2 The goniometer

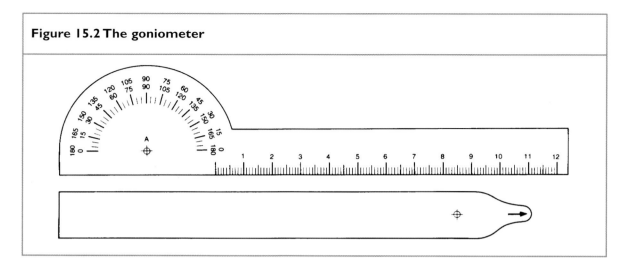

centres of rotation for the large joints. To maintain accuracy, the arms of the goniometer must be positioned parallel to the bones along the mid-line of the limb. Figures 15.3(a) and 15.3(b) show correct and incorrect alignment respectively. In figure 15.3(b), the upper arm of the goniometer is not aligned along the mid-line of the upper leg, so the reading obtained is lower, giving the appearance of a less flexible joint.

Accuracy in measurements

Spine and hip movement

When the spine is moving in combination with either the lower limb or upper limb, close examination is required to determine which joints are actually taking part in the stretching exercise. Tightness in the ligaments surrounding the hip means that, once the hip has flexed beyond 90 degrees, the pelvis starts to tilt and the lower spine subsequently begins to flex. Total range of motion may be made up of movements at a number of joints. In figure 15.4(a), the individual appears to have long hamstrings because he is able to touch his toes. In fact, the hamstrings are short and the pelvis has stayed tilted back. The movement is occurring in the lumbar spine because the individual's spinal extensors are excessively flexible. In figure 15.4(b), the hamstrings are also short like those of the individual in 15.4(a), but the spinal extensors are of average length so the total range of motion is considerably reduced. In figure 15.4(c), the range of motion appears normal, but neither the hamstrings nor

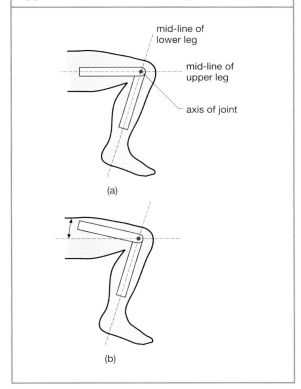

Figure 15.3 Correct goniometer position: (a) correct alignment of goniometre with arms along mid-line of limb; (b) incorrect alignment gives appearance of reduced range of motion

mid-line of
lower leg

mid-line of
upper leg

axis of joint

(a)

(b)

the spinal extensors is flexible. Instead, the movement is coming from the thoracic spine, which is rounding excessively.

Pelvic and hip movement

Pelvic tilt is also an important factor in determining hip motion. In figures 15.5(a) and 15.5(b), the length of the rectus femoris is being measured. In figure 15.5(a), no pelvic tilt is occurring and the range of hip extension is seen to be limited. In figure 15.5(b), the same range of hip

extension is occurring, but the anterior tilt of the pelvis, occurring at the same time, gives the appearance of an increase in total range of motion.

Spine and shoulder movement

Movement of the spine with the shoulder is also important. In figures 15.6(a) and 15.6(b), the range of shoulder elevation is being measured against the wall. In figure 15.6(a), the movement is seen to be limited, but in figure 15.6(b) there appears to be a greater range of motion. In fact, the range of motion at the shoulder is exactly the same in each case; it is the movement occurring in the spine that is greater in the second figure.

When measuring joint movement, it is essential to limit the motion to a single joint. This can be achieved by looking closely at the body and repeating the movement to ensure accuracy.

Using flexibility measures in research studies

When flexibility measures are being used as part of a research study, as discussed in Chapter 6, we need to be sure that the tests are both accurate and giving us the information that we think they are. Although a full discussion of experimental design and research techniques is not within the scope of this book, we will look at some fundamental processes. The interested reader is referred to Thomas and Nelson (1990) for further information.

Validity and *reliability* are two essential factors in measurement error. Validity asks the question, 'Does the test measure what it claims to do?', whereas reliability asks, 'Was each test of a batch the same?' Both are essential for maintaining the accuracy of stretching tests.

Figure 15.4 Sit-and-reach test – what is being measured? (a) excessive flexibility in spinal extensions; (b) excessive rounding of thoracic spine; (c) normal back flexion and short hamstrings

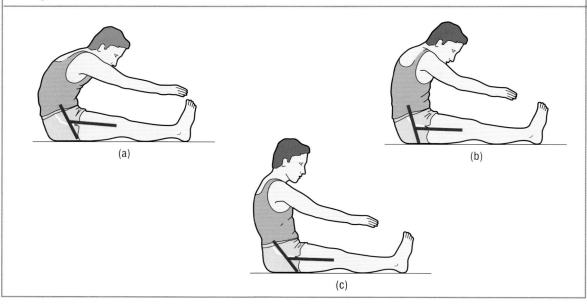

(a) (b) (c)

Figure 15.5 Pelvic tilt and hip extension

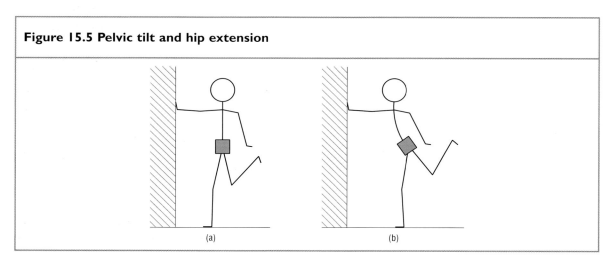

(a) (b)

Key point: Validity asks, 'Does the test measure what we think it does?'; reliability asks, 'Was each test really the same?'

Validity

Take the example of a straight leg raise (SLR) action to measure hamstring length. We perform

Figure 15.6 Spine and shoulder movements

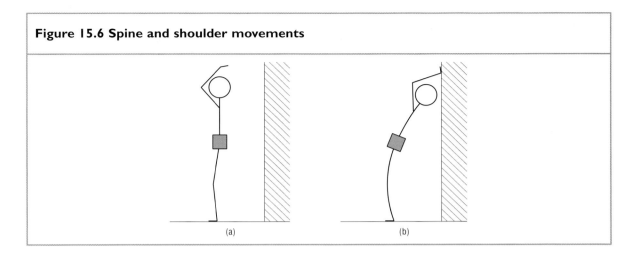

(a) (b)

a certain number of stretches over six weeks and use the SLR to determine the best number of stretches for increasing hamstring flexibility. Is this a valid measure?

There are two types of validity: internal and external. *Internal validity* refers to the extent to which the results of a study can be attributed to the exercises (intervention) used. For example, if flexibility on the SLR does increase after six weeks, was this the result of our stretching programme or something else such as simply the passage of time? *External validity* is concerned with the generalisation of the results. In other words, are the changes that occurred in our experiment likely to occur outside the laboratory situation? Sometimes, an experiment may be so controlled that it no longer reflects what occurs in sport. For example, if we choose to measure the SLR lying flat and using a frame that fixes the pelvis and prevent the knee from bending to ensure accuracy, how does this compare to a football-kicking action where the hamstrings are stretched in sport? Clearly, there may be so many differences that the exercise is no longer the same as the functional action.

Internal validity

A number of factors may affect internal validity.

- **History** can affect internal validity if some other event occurred at the same time as testing that could have affected the results. For example, if we used students for our experimental subjects, some of them may have started a gymnastic programme at school at the same time as the experiment, and they may well have used hamstring stretching as part of their gymnastics. This makes it impossible to say whether our study, or the gymnastics, was responsible for any results obtained.

- **Maturation** refers to the passage of time. This is important when a study, especially with children, lasts for a prolonged period. For example, if we have a group of ten-year-olds and our study lasts for 2–3 years, are any results simply the effect of moving into adolescence and the flexibility changes that occur during this time?

- **Testing** will itself affect the results. Once we have measured hamstring length using the SLR, we have in fact stretched the hamstrings with the SLR test. The subjects have

Table 15.1   Flexibility tests

Tick ( ) the box corresponding to your movement range following the guidelines listed below.

- Perform thorough warm-up before measuring your flexibility
- Hold each stretched position for three seconds before measuring
- Do not bounce into the movement
- Average values will vary with body-size and body-type

Test	Poor	Average	Good
Keep your straight leg on the floor and pull your bent knee towards your chest	knee further than 15 cm from rib-cage	knee 10–15 cm from rib-cage	knee to rib-cage
Keep the soles of your feet together and press your knees downwards towards the floor	more than 15cm from floor	15 cm from floor	less than 15 cm from floor
Keep the knees locked and reach forwards towards the toes	more than 15cm from toes	10–15 cm from toes	touching toes

Table 15.1	Flexibility tests cont.		
Test	Poor	Average	Good
The lower leg is bent up to the chest and held still, the top leg lowers towards the ground	above horizontal	horizontal	below horizontal
Stand 0.5m from a wall. Lean forwards, keeping the feet flat on the floor and the knees locked	more than 60 degrees	60 degrees	less than 60 degrees
Keep the forehead and chest on the ground and lift the straight arm upwards	less than 15 cm	15–20 cm	more than 20 cm

Table 15.1	Flexibility tests cont.		
Test	Poor	Average	Good
Reach behind the back and try to grip the fingers of the opposite hand	fingers more than 15 cm apart	fingers 10–15 cm apart	fingers touching
Keep the arms straight and try to cross them over as far as possible	cross at wrist	cross at elbow	cross at upper arm
Keep the foot flat on a stool and press the knee towards the wall	more than 50 degrees	40–50 degrees	less than 40 degrees

Table 15.1	Flexibility tests cont.		
Test	Poor	Average	Good
Keep the knees together and bent to 90 degrees. Allow the heels to drop outwards	less than 70 degrees	70–90 degrees	more than 90 degrees
Lock the arms flat out and measure the distance between the pelvic crest and the floor	more than 15 cm	15–10 cm	less than 5 cm
Keep the arms flat on the floor and twist the trunk to allow the knees to lower towards the floor	more than 10 cm	10 cm	0 cm

Table 15.1	Flexibility tests cont.			
Test		**Poor**	**Average**	**Good**
Keep the small of the back on the chair back and flex the spine (not the hips) maximally		fingers to mid-shin	fingers to floor	flat hand to floor
Keep the feet flat and the knees locked. Without leaning forwards or backwards reach down the side of the leg		fingers above knee	fingers to knee	fingers below knee
Keep both legs straight and flex one hip as far as possible		less than 90 degrees	90 degrees	more than 90 degrees

Table 15.1	Flexibility tests cont.		
Test	**Poor**	**Average**	**Good**
Abduct both legs while keeping the small of the back flat and the legs straight	less than 90 degrees	90 degrees	more than 90 degrees
Keep the knees together and flex one knee maximally	knee further than 10 cm from buttock	knee 5–10 cm from buttock	knee to buttock
Keep the knees and ankles together throughout the test. Slowly sit back on to the heels. Measure the distance between the top (dorsum) of the foot and the ground	greater than 5 cm	5 cm	flat

learned how to perform the test, and may be able to relax their muscles further.

- **Instrumentation** changes are also very important. For example, if we are using a goniometer (*see* page 196), the position of the goniometer and the type of goniometer used must remain the same; otherwise, the measurement obtained will be different, not through stretching, but through inaccurate measurement.
- **Statistical regression** is a tendency for factors to vary, especially if extreme measures (very flexible or very inflexible) are used. If we choose a group with very tight hamstrings for our study, we would expect them to vary in such a way as to move towards the average score. This is because all scores will vary with each measurement; sometimes a person is more flexible, and sometimes less. We are only measuring an average for that individual, and that average will constantly change.
- **Selection biases** encompass the number of factors involved in picking subjects for the study in the first place. For example, if we ask for volunteers for a flexibility study, we may well get a lot of individuals who think they are flexible (we all like to show off!). Equally, those who stay with the study (six weeks is a long time) are likely to be those who are enjoying it, or have a particular reason to do it (perhaps it is a requirement for their college course).

External validity

When dealing with threats to external validity, remember that we are concerned with whether our results accurately reflect what happens in the real world.

- If we use a pre-test, i.e. we allow an individual to get used to the experimental setup before we test them, we may get **reactive effects of testing**. The subject would be prepared for the test and aware of what was coming. This would not occur on the sports field, for example, where the stretch would be performed during an exercise.
- We must also be careful that the way we select individuals for our study does not **interact** with the measurement we are using. For example, test results from subjects who know where their hamstrings are may differ from subjects who do not have this knowledge.
- If the results of our testing only occur in the laboratory but not in the real world, we are seeing **reactive effects of the experimental setup**. For example, we may choose to take a measurement with a very complex piece of apparatus that influences movement to such a degree that the movement is no longer similar to the one used in sport.
- If two or more stretches are given, the effects of one exercise may influence the other, and we have **multiple treatment interference**.

> **Key point**: *Internal validity* asks whether the results of a study are really due to the stretching exercises used (known as the 'intervention'. *External validity* asks whether the results obtained in a laboratory experiment actually mirror the results that would have occurred in the real world.

Reliability

Reliability is really the consistency of the results obtained from a series of tests. We can talk about reliability in terms of *observed score, true score and error score*. When we measure range of motion with a goniometer, for example, we are not measuring the real joint angle, because the goniometer is attached to the skin and not to the bones. What we are seeing is an *observed* score. If we were to x-ray the moving joint and measure the bones directly, we would obtain the *true score*. The difference between these two,

Table 15.2

Landmark	Position
• Lateral malleolus of tibia	• Outside bone of ankle
• Head of the fibula	• Outside bone of knee splint bone
• Lateral epicondlyle of femur	• Outside upper knee
• Greater trochanter	• Outside upper thigh/hip
• Anterior superior iliac spine	• Point on outside/upper pelvis
• Posterior superior iliac spine	• Dimple at upper tail bone
• Acromion process	• Point at end of collar bone

the real range of motion and the apparent range of motion, is the *error* score.

The error in a measurement may come from four main sources.

- **Subject** errors include things such as motivation, fatigue and health. If, in our study, an individual injures their hamstrings, this will affect their flexibility and, therefore, the test results. Equally, a subject who is less motivated may not pull the limb as far as they would if they were practising an active stretch.
- **Test** errors may occur through lack of practice and familiarity with the results, for example, as well as through technique and lack of attention to detail. When a tester knows the value of a result, they may be able to influence it by over- or under-estimating a measurement. Equally, a poor standard of testing through lax positioning of a goniometer, for example, may produce considerable error.
- **Scoring** error is due to the selection of inappropriate measurement values, for example measuring joint movement in single inches rather than degrees.
- **Instrumentation** error results when instruments are not calibrated, or they simply break down – something that happens all too often.

Reliability and testers

An additional aspect of reliability concerns the variation of the results obtained for a test from day to day, or between two people performing the same test. This is especially important if we are using a test to measure progress or to assess the effectiveness of a particular fitness or rehabilitation programme. For example, if tester A measures the flexibility of a subject's hamstrings using a straight leg raise (SLR) test today, will they use *exactly* the same test when they test again tomorrow, or next week? This is called *intra-tester* (or *intra-rater*) *reliability*, and is a measure of the consistency or repeatability of a particular measure. The more complex a test, the less reliable it is likely to be, because it will be easier to make mistakes when applying the test. Alternatively, tester A uses the SLR test to measure a subject's hamstring flexibility, and for the next workout tester B uses the same test on the same subject, are both testers applying the test in exactly the same way? This is called *inter-tester* (*inter-rater*) *reliability*.

To improve both intra- and inter-tester reliability, the tests that we use should be agreed by everyone so that we all apply them in the same way. Also, if we are measuring parts of the body, it is better to base our measurements on bone rather than skin and muscle (soft tissue), as bone is less likely to change or vary. Soft tissue can swell, build up with strength training, waste with disuse etc., whereas bone will not. For this reason, we use the pieces of bone that are close to the skin's surface as the points to measure. These are called 'bony landmarks', and some are listed in table 15.2.

Summary

- We need to measure flexibility to know the current level of a client's movement range.
- Measuring flexibility enables us to judge if any muscle imbalance exists, and to chart a client's progress.
- Flexibility can be measured using score charts, measuring devices (goniometers) and photographs.
- Angles obtained during measurement are compared to normal values and to the other side of the client's body.
- Measurements may appear accurate when, in fact, they are not. Exercises that combine movements of two body-parts simultaneously must be checked closely.
- Validity asks, 'Does a test measure what it claims to do?', while reliability asks, 'Was each test of a batch the same?'

16

STRETCHING AND SPORTS INJURIES

Tissue healing

If you slip on a pavement and sprain your ankle, your body reacts immediately by starting a healing process. This process can be divided into three phases: *inflammation*, *proliferation* (sometimes called regeneration), and *remodelling*.

Inflammation

Following injury, the inflammatory phase lasts between four and six days. The appearance of the body at this time reveals four classic signs: redness, swelling, heat and pain, which together lead to a loss of function in the injured bodypart (*see* fig 16.1).

- **Redness**: When tissues tear, small blood vessels are ruptured, releasing blood into the surrounding area. Injured tissue-cells die and chemicals are released, irritating the local tissues and causing local blood flow to increase. This leads to the red appearance.
- **Swelling**: Changes in the concentration of

fluids around the blood vessels cause watery fluid to leak out of them and into the surrounding tissues, giving rise to swelling. If the injury is close to the body surface, for example an injured ankle ligament, the swelling is readily apparent; if the injury is deeper in, however, the swelling may not be seen on the body surface, but only felt as pressure and stiffness.

- **Heat**: Increased metabolic activity from the inflammation causes heat, which is felt over the skin surface.
- **Pain**: The combination of pressure from the swelling and chemical irritation from metabolic products causes pain.

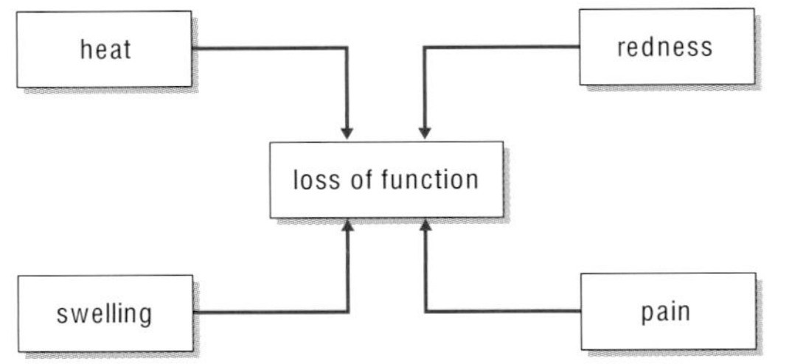

With a minor injury, the inflammatory phase may end in three days, but with more serious injuries, inflammation can remain active for five or six days. When an injury occurs and the tissues tear, their tensile strength (capacity to stretch) immediately drops (*see* fig 16.2). During the inflammatory phase, the strength of the injured tissues relies on clotted blood and tissue fluids, so the injured area is very weak. Until the blood and swelling clears and new collagen tissue forms (*see* below), the tensile strength of the area remains poor. During this time, we say that the tissues are in their 'lag' phase where, although healing is progressing, tissue strength remains unaltered. Any stretching applied at this stage can easily disrupt the healing process and prolong the inflammation, making the total healing time longer.

Figure 16.1 The signs of inflammation

heat → loss of function ← redness

swelling → loss of function ← pain

Key point: The time from injury occurring to the beginning of the formation of strong collagen, which bridges the injured area, is about three to five days. Do not stretch before this time as the tissues are too weak.

Proliferation

Following inflammation, *proliferation* occurs. Within the injured area, the cells that were supplied by the damaged blood capillaries will have died, and these must be removed if healing is to be effective. Removal of dead cells is the job of special blood cells that engulf the dead material and digest it. Once this has occurred, new capillaries start to grow into the damaged area, forming delicate granulation tissue. By the third to fifth day after injury, a special form of tissue called *collagen* (see page 21) has started to form; this material will join the damaged tissues by forming a 'bridge'.

The collagen fibres are laid down haphazardly and, if this orientation remains, the scar formed will be very weak. To improve the strength of the scar, gentle movement should be performed, which will stretch the healing collagen fibres and cause them to line up in the direction of stress applied, making the eventual scar far stronger. The size of the collagen fibres also depends on regular movement: with exercise, larger and stronger fibres form and the fibres bond to each other, further increasing the tissue strength. Exercise, correctly prescribed, will therefore create a stronger and more suitable healing breach across injured tissues (this is represented by the dotted line on the graph shown in figure 16.2). Most of the collagen will have been laid

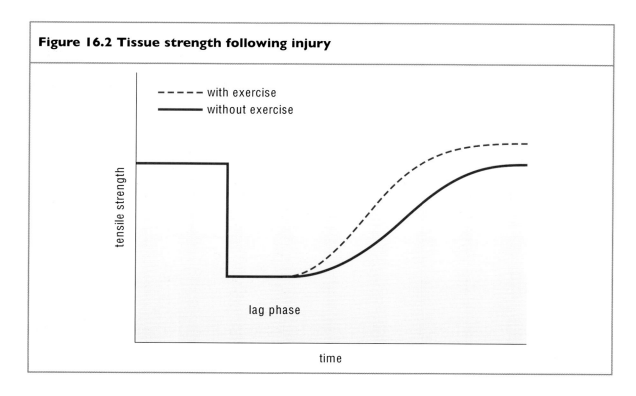

Figure 16.2 Tissue strength following injury

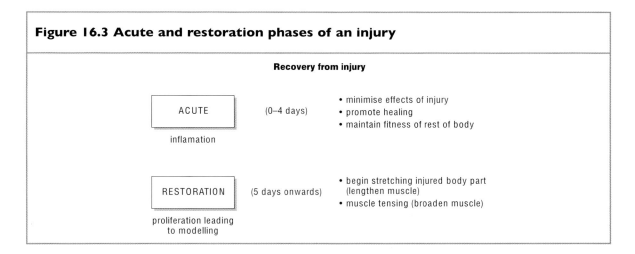

Figure 16.3 Acute and restoration phases of an injury

Recovery from injury

ACUTE (0–4 days)
inflamation

• minimise effects of injury
• promote healing
• maintain fitness of rest of body

RESTORATION (5 days onwards)
proliferation leading to modelling

• begin stretching injured body part (lengthen muscle)
• muscle tensing (broaden muscle)

down by 16 to 21 days after injury, so this is the time when stiffness will be greatest and stretching will be most effective.

> **Key point**: Gentle exercise strengthens the collagen tissue bridge, which forms as part of the healing process.

Remodelling

About 21 days after the injury, the *remodelling* phase begins. During this phase, the amount of collagen produced is equal to the amount broken down. Although the total amount of collagen remains the same, the fibres overlap and form a mat of adhesions, which will stick to the surrounding tissues if movement is not performed. The collagen will also begin to shrink unless stretching exercises are continued. The function of this phase of healing is to make the healing bridge as similar as possible to the tissue that was injured. Although the tissue bridge will not look exactly like the injured tissue, its function will be similar. For this reason, exercise is vital. Without exercise, the bridge ends up tight and short, restricting normal movements and sometimes causing changes in alignment.

Time-scale for stretching

As we discussed above, it is clear from the effect on healing that stretching is not appropriate immediately after injury for the following two reasons. First, the injured area is very weak and easily disrupted. Any amount of stretching could easily pull it and increase the tissue damage, which in turn will re-start the inflammation. Second, collagen tissue will not begin to form until the dead material produced by the injury is removed, so until that happens there is nothing there to stretch. We can divide the post-injury period into two distinct phases (*see* fig 16.3).

Acute phase

The first is the *acute* phase, from the day of injury to three or four days after. During this time the area is still inflamed, and our aim should be to minimise the effects of the injury. This can be achieved by using ice or cold water to slow down the metabolic rate (the amount of tissue activity), and reduce cell death from the low amount of oxygen present in the area. Swelling should be contained by using an elasticated bandage, and the fitness of the rest of the body should be maintained by using exercises that do not stress the injured area.

Restoration phase

After four or five days the inflammation will have subsided, and we enter the *restoration* phase. Stretching is needed to ensure that the collagen fibres of the injured tissue strengthen and face in the right direction to support the body-part. Strengthening exercises must also be performed to tense and broaden the muscles. This moves the muscle fibres apart and prevents them from sticking together.

> **Key point**: In the acute phase of an injury, use cold water or ice and an elasticated bandage to limit swelling and further tissue damage. In the restorative phase, use both stretching and strengthening to lengthen and broaden the tissues.

Classification of injury

When muscles are injured, we say they are *strained*; when ligaments are injured, they are *sprained*. Both strains and sprains can be categorised into grades that represent the severity of the injury and the amount of tissue that has been damaged.

Ligament injuries (sprains)

Three grades of ligament injuries are used. Grade I sprains involve only slight tissue damage and the area is tender to touch, swelling is only slight and the body-part moves almost normally. With grade II sprains, more ligament fibres are injured, local pain is more intense and movement is more limited. Grade I and II injuries are common when, for example, the ankle is twisted. Grade III injuries are far more serious because they involve complete rupture of the tendon. A skiing injury is a typical example of this type. There is considerable pain and swelling, and it is impossible to take the body-weight through the injured limb. These injuries often require surgery to repair the ruptured ligament, followed by intensive physiotherapy.

Muscle injuries (strains)

Muscle strains can be classified into four grades. Grade I (mild) strains involve tearing of only a few muscle fibres and subsequent local bruising. The area feels stiff for a few days and then clears up fairly quickly. Grade II (moderate) strains are more severe. A larger number of muscle fibres are injured, and injury occurs over a greater area. The muscle membrane (fascia) still remains intact, so bleeding is contained within the muscle and forms what is called an *intramuscular haematoma*. The area again feels tight, but this time a local raised area is felt over the bruising and the muscle gives pain when tensed or stretched. A pulled hamstring is an example of a grade I or II muscle strain. With grade III (severe) strains, a larger area of muscle is affected. The muscle fascia is partially torn, and more than one muscle may be involved. Bleeding is more profuse, and it spreads over a larger area: because the muscle fascia has torn, blood spreads throughout the area, causing skin discoloration. A typical example here is a 'dead leg', where bruising spreads from the injured thigh down into the knee and calf. The grade IV injury is a complete rupture. The muscle-ends contract and a distinct gap can be felt between the injured muscle fibres. In some cases, a snapping sound may have been heard at the time of injury. Bleeding and swelling are considerable, and the muscle cannot be tensed up. This type of injury may require hospital treatment.

The classification of an injury is a guide to the period of rest and the amount of stretching that is required. As a general rule, the stretching should not be painful, but you should feel that it is lengthening the muscle. Never force a stretch, and never exercise through increasing pain. If something is painful, and the pain goes away with stretching, that is fine. However, if the pain starts to increase, the stretch should be stopped.

> **Key point**: Never exercise through increasing pain. If something hurts and the pain eases with exercise, it is safe to continue. If the pain gets worse, stop immediately.

Stretching exercises for injuries

The following stretches are for general guidance only. If you suffer a sports injury, see a physiotherapist. The sooner an injury is seen, the better; if left without treatment, injuries can put you out of sport for far longer. In addition, minor aches and pains are often signs that something is going wrong with the body. If this is caught in time, a more severe injury can often be prevented.

The sprained ankle

When you sprain your ankle, the most common injury is to a portion of the lateral ligament on the outside of the joint. This tissue limits plantarflexion, inversion and adduction of the foot. The easiest way to stretch this area is to cross the injured leg at the shin over the uninjured one; one hand steadies the lower leg on the injured side, while the other is cupped around the foot and ankle to pull it down, round and inwards. The stretch should be gentle and static.

Once this has been achieved, the next stage is to stretch the ankle actively by standing and rocking over on to the outer edge of the foot, or by walking on an inclined surface. This movement is controlled, but eventually faster actions must be used to develop agility in the ankle structures. This can be achieved by walking on an uneven surface such as soft ground or sand.

You can also make your own uneven surface by placing four or five cushions on the ground and walking, and then slowly jogging, over them in bare feet. At each stage, the action must be controlled so you don't feel that the movement is 'running away' with you.

As well as stretching the side of the ankle, walking on a uneven surface also strengthens the muscles surrounding the ankle so that they can support or 'stabilise' the joint. This function of ankle stability is the most important aspect of fitness to develop following an injury. Another way to work on stability of this type is to stand on one leg (the injured one) and hold this position for 20–30 seconds. When you do this, you will notice all of the muscles around the ankle 'flickering' as they work hard to stabilise the joint.

> **Key point**: Following a sprained ankle, stretch the outside of the joint using a plantarflexion and inversion movement and stabilise the joint using single-leg standing.

Shin splints

Shin splints is a condition affecting the shin muscles, which are contained within compartments running alongside the tibia and fibula.

215

With training, the muscles swell and thicken and, as this happens, the pressure within them increases. Because the muscles are contained within an inflexible compartment, they cannot bulge outwards; therefore, they bulge inwards, cutting off their own blood supply. It is this reduction of blood flow and the build-up of acids within the muscles that causes pain. Stretching exercises can help some types of shin splints by preventing the muscles becoming short and tight.

On the front of the shin, the the anterior compartment contains tibialis anterior and the toe extensors (*see* fig 16.4). These muscles pull the foot and toes up into dorsiflexion. To stretch them, we have to press the foot slowly into plantarflexion immediately after running (*see* exercise 17). We begin by kneeling with the feet flat on the ground. From this position we sit back onto the heels, pressing the feet into plantarflexion. To increase the stretch on the toes, place a folded towel on the floor beneath the toes to press them into flexion. Hold the position for 30–60 seconds to allow the muscles to 'give' gradually. Repeat the stretch five times after each run.

The pulled hamstring

When you tear a hamstring, you may injure the muscle in its centre part (belly) or at the musculo-tendinous (MT) junction – the point at which the hamstring joins to the bones of the pelvis, or the knee, via the muscle tendon (*see* fig 16.5). The difference between these two areas is that the MT junction does not contract, while the muscle belly does. As well as stretching, muscle-belly tears will need strength training to broaden the muscle and separate the muscle fibres to prevent them sticking together. Injury to the MT junction often responds to stretching alone.

Figure 16.4 Compartments of the lower leg (Norris 1998)

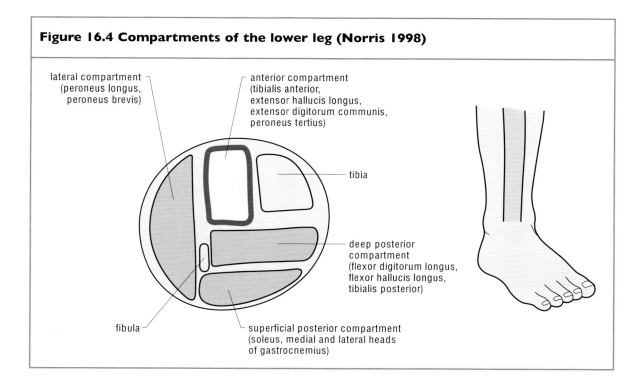

lateral compartment
(peroneus longus,
peroneus brevis)

anterior compartment
(tibialis anterior,
extensor hallucis longus,
extensor digitorum communis,
peroneus tertius)

tibia

deep posterior
compartment
(flexor digitorum longus,
flexor hallucis longus,
tibialis posterior)

fibula

superficial posterior compartment
(soleus, medial and lateral heads
of gastrocnemius)

Figure 16.5 Areas of injury in a muscle

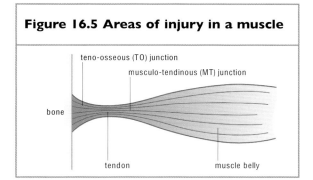

Figure 16.6 Combining strength and stretch of the hamstrings: (a) hip extension over side of bench; (b) combined knee and hip extension against partner's resistance; (c) sprint jumping.

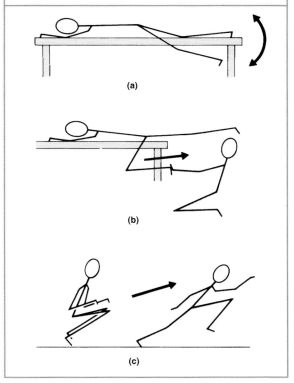

Because the hamstrings work over the hip and the knee, two types of stretches are necessary. First, the muscle must be stretched with the leg straight (*see* exercise 29). Then, once adequate flexibility has been regained, the elastic strength of the muscle must be worked on. First stretch the muscle, then contract it rapidly from this lengthened position. To do this, lie face-down on a bench with the injured leg over the bench side so that the hip is flexed to 90 degrees. A small (3 kg) weight is attached around the ankle. From the stretched position, the hip is extended to pull the leg upwards against the resistance of the weight (*see* fig 16.6(a)). The movement can be modified to use both the knee and the hip by training with a partner. The partner provides the resistance by pushing on the heel, and the movement starts with the knee and hip both flexed to 90 degrees. From here, extend both the hip and knee simultaneously against resistance, hold the maximally contracted position for one to two seconds, and then lower the leg while maintaining tension in the muscle (*see* fig 16.6(b)). This controlled action progresses to spring jumping actions (*see* fig 16.6(c)), moving from a flexed hip/knee position to a fully extended position.

To work the upper part of the hamstrings and the gluteals, we have to perform a posterior pelvic tilt against resistance. Functionally, the action involves lifting, so this can become a useful exercise. The action is called a 'hip hinge' or 'good morning' exercise (*see* fig 16.7). Begin by standing with your legs straight and a stick across the shoulders. Keeping the legs and back straight, bend forwards from the hips to 45 degrees, and then return to standing. The action must move from the hip as a pivot rather than from the lumbar spine: moving from the lumbar spine will dangerously overstretch the lumbar tissues.

In sport, the hamstring muscles work with a 'whipping' action, often stretching rapidly. In

Figure 16.7 Hip hinge action

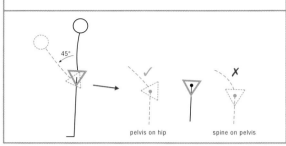

order to be sport-specific, our stretching programme must reflect this, so dynamic stretching (*see* page 58) is required. For this, exercise 122 (Leg swing – forwards and backwards) is used. Swing the leg progressively to shin, waist and then chest level, beginning slowly and gradually building up speed. Once you are confident with this single plane (flexion–extension) action, change to a multi-plane movement, kicking across the body (extension–abduction to flexion–adduction) and build in rotation movements. The final stage of progression is to use sports actions (such as kicking a football) as exercise. Begin with a slow gentle tap and build to a rapid kick, aiming to cover a large distance.

> **Key point**: The hamstrings perform fast whipping actions in sport and work over two joints. Begin with slow static stretching and build to dynamic stretching, using single- and two-joint activities.

The swollen knee

When the knee suffers a minor injury, it will swell and limit the movement of the joint. As the swelling clots and the injury heals, both the physiological movements and the accessory movements of the joint will be limited. This means that the joint will lose its normal movement and its healthy springy feeling (joint play). Stretching into flexion and extension will help you to regain the physiological movements, but the accessory movements will only return if these actions are combined with stresses to the knee that apply rotatory and shearing forces. These will work on all aspects of agility, and also help to build 'confidence' in the knee.

Start by standing with the feet shoulder width apart, then step forwards and across with the uninjured leg so that the stress is taken on the injured knee. Step backwards and across to place the opposite stress on the joint (*see* fig 16.8(a)). This action can be used as a side-step to perform a 'grapevine' action. Bending the knee further will increase the stress on the knee, and performing the action over a bench to bend the knee to near maximum will test the knee fully (*see* fig 16.8(b)). Because these actions stress the knee considerably, they must be carefully controlled.

When the rotation movement of the knee is limited, particularly after injury to the inner ligament (medial collateral ligament), this can be regained by twisting the tibia on the femur. A simple exercise is to place the foot up on a swivel chair so that the knee and hip are flexed to 90 degrees. Turn the chair by twisting the tibia and foot. As the foot moves outwards, the tibia is externally rotated and the medial ligament is stretched. Gentle stretching of this type will make the ligament stronger by stressing and relaxing it to help the ligament fibres line up in the direction of the stress on the knee.

The 'kicking' muscle

Injury to the rectus femoris or the 'kicking muscle' is common in football. The injury usually occurs either when an ineffective warm-up has been performed, or towards the end of the

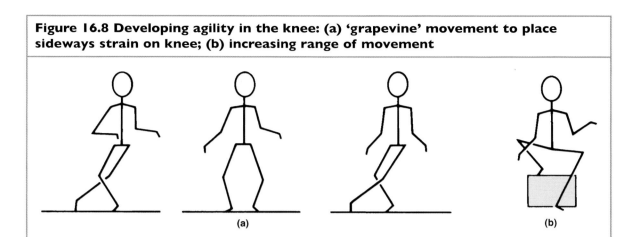

Figure 16.8 Developing agility in the knee: (a) 'grapevine' movement to place sideways strain on knee; (b) increasing range of movement

(a)

(b)

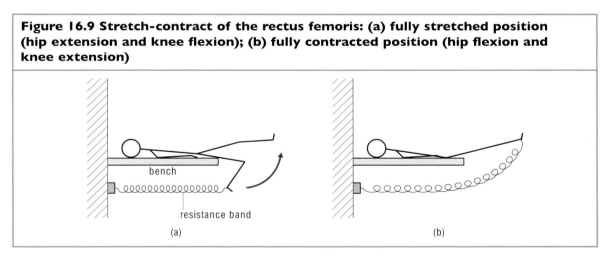

Figure 16.9 Stretch-contract of the rectus femoris: (a) fully stretched position (hip extension and knee flexion); (b) fully contracted position (hip flexion and knee extension)

bench

resistance band

(a)

(b)

game when fatigue sets in. Either way, stretching is needed to restore the length and spring of the muscle. Passive stretching is performed by simultaneously flexing the knee and extending the hip. Once the same range can be achieved on both the injured and the uninjured side, the elastic strength of the muscle must be worked on. The action is to move from a fully stretched position to a fully contracted position of hip flexion and knee extension. This is performed against a resistance which can be supplied by an elastic band, by a low pulley in a weight training room or by a training partner (*see* fig 16.9).

Groin strain

Groin strain is also a common injury in football, as well as in other sports that involve rapid sideways stretches of 45° or greater while lunging or side-stepping. The adductor muscles of the hip attach to the lower part of the pelvis. The adductor longus, adductor magnus and adductor brevis all attach to the femur and have no action over the knee; the gracilis, however, attaches to the upper part of the inner surface of the tibia, so it can also flex the knee during certain actions. This is important, because adductor stretches must be performed both with the knee flexed to take the gracilis off stretch and tax the other adductors, and with the knee extended to stretch the gracilis itself. Two exercises are useful.

In the first exercise (*see* fig 16.10(a)), begin by sitting on the floor with the soles of the feet together. Holding the feet with the hands, press down on to the knees or thighs to force them into abduction.

The second stretch emphasises the gracilis. For this, lie on the back with the legs straight. Flex the right leg to 90 degrees at the hips, keeping it straight. From this position the leg is abducted, aiming to rest it on the floor (*see* fig 16.10(b)). Repeat using the left leg. In both exercises, PNF (contract–relax) stretching may be performed by lifting the legs against resistance (manual in the first stretch, gravity in the second) and then lowering the legs again to increase the range of motion. It is important for total rehabilitation of the adductor muscles following groin strain that strength training and stretching go hand in hand.

Figure 16.10(a) Hip adductor stretch for groin strain

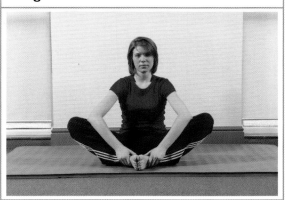

Figure 16.10(b) Hip adductor stretch for groin strain

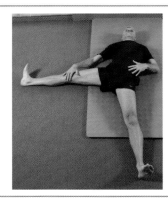

As the rehabilitation period progresses, fast explosive actions (plyometrics) must be built in. This can be done usefully in a swimming pool with breaststroke type actions and using elastic tubing in the gym. In addition, jogging, cutting, side stepping and zigzag running drills constitute dynamic stretching and also prepare the muscle with sport-specific actions.

> **Key point**: Following a groin injury, static stretches should be performed both with the knee bent and with it straight. Static stretches should then be progressed to dynamic stretching, plyometrics and running drills.

Clicking hip and clicking knee

Clicking hip and clicking knee are two conditions that can result from tightness in the ilio-tibial band (ITB), the strong band of fascia that runs along the outside of the leg (*see* fig 16.11). At its top, the ITB attaches to the hip muscles and then passes over a knobble of bone at the top of the thighbone (femur) called the greater trochanter. As the leg is moved forwards and backwards, the ITB passes in front and behind the trochanter. If tight, the ITB will flick over the trochanter like a guitar string. This causes pain and swelling, and often a clicking sensation that can be felt and, in extreme cases, actually heard. A similar mechanism exists at the knee, where the ITB can flick over a point of bone on the lower end of the thighbone called the lateral epicondyle. The painful clicking sensation that occurs here is often called 'runners knee'.

To reduce the chance of these conditions occurring, or to lessen the pain if they already exist, ITB stretching is used. Exercise 32 is designed to stretch the ITB by holding the pelvis still and adducting the hip. The position is held for 30–40 seconds, and initially only three reps are used. The movement should be performed daily.

The upper portion of the ITB at the hip may be isolated using exercise 31. Again, the pelvis is held still while the hip is adducted. This time,

however, the knee is bent, releasing the stretch in the lower portion of the ITB and throwing greater stress on the upper portion.

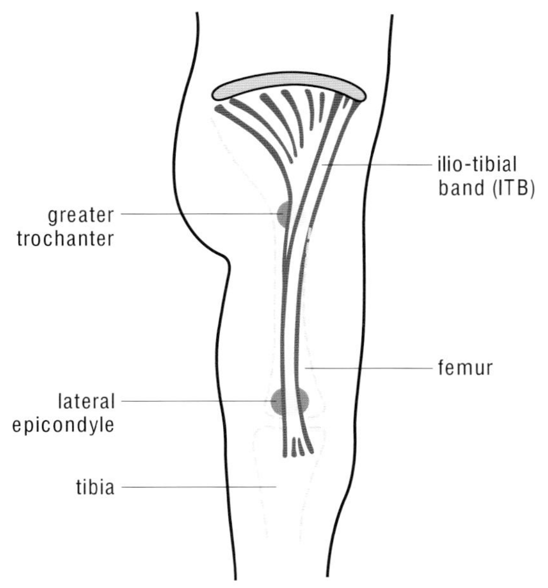

The dead leg

A 'dead leg' occurs when the quadriceps muscles of the thigh are severely bruised. This normally happens in rugby when a knee or head contacts the thigh at speed in a tackle. Blood vessels are ruptured and a large amount of blood is released into the muscle. The result is a large tense area within the muscle caused by a combination of blood and swelling. As the condition heals, the bruising tracks down through the muscle into the knee and calf. The athlete is unable to bend the knee because of tension in the quadriceps. The danger with this injury is that the release of blood can cause the area to calcify and form calcium bone salts within the muscle. If this happens it can be very serious, so stretching must be applied very cautiously under the supervision of a physiotherapist.

Initially, only active stretches should be used by lying on your front and simply flexing the knee through the power of the hamstrings alone. Once 90-degree knee flexion has been obtained, very gentle passive stretches can be performed by lying on your back and pulling the heel up towards the buttock. A towel placed around the ankle makes the reach easier. When the range of movement increases further and the pain and bruising subside, greater overpressure can be used to stretch the quadriceps by kneeling and sitting back on the ankles. These quadriceps stretches are described in Chapter 7, exercises 17 and 30.

Figure 16.11 The ilio-tibial band (ITB)

ilio-tibial band (ITB)

greater trochanter

femur

lateral epicondyle

tibia

The calf and Achilles

When the Achilles is injured, calf stretches should be performed with the knee flexed (*see* exercise 9); when the calf is injured, it is usually the long gastrocnemius muscle that is affected, and this should be stretched with the knee straight. When this can be performed statically without pain, the following active stretch is used.

Stand on a 5 cm block (a thick book) and place the ball of the foot on the back edge. Allow the heel to lower down, keeping the knee locked: this will stretch the gastrocnemius. Starting from the standing position again, raise up on to the toes against your body-weight. Initially, you should hold on to something to take some of your body-weight off the calf. Eventually, full body-weight can be used and the exercise can be speeded up until faster, more explosive actions are used to work the muscle for elastic strength.

The arch of the foot

In sports such as the martial arts and some types of dance, which are carried out in bare feet or in very thin shoes, the amount of motion available to the big toe joint can overstretch one of the structures that forms the arch of the foot. This structure, the *plantarfascia*, can become inflamed or damaged. If this happens, stretching should be employed once the injury has healed in order to restore flexibility. This can be achieved by plantarflexing the foot and flexing the toes simultaneously (*see* exercise 38). The plantarfascia will stand out as a tight cord in the sole of the foot.

The ribs

The ribs can be bruised or cracked, for example in a rugby tackle or when hit by the ball in hockey or cricket. When the injury has healed, stiffness often remains because the muscles between the ribs (intercostals) have tightened. To open the ribs and stretch the intercostals, we need to combine overhead reaching actions with deep breathing. Twisting the trunk away from the painful area will increase the stretch still further. When performing this exercise, be careful not to take too many deep breaths without a rest, because this could cause you to hyperventilate and become light-headed. Perform the exercise three times and then breathe normally for 30–60 seconds before trying again.

The frozen shoulder

When the shoulder is injured, it will swell and the joint capsule will fill with fluid. This will cause the capsule to tighten, eventually limiting the movement of the whole joint. Due to the shape of the capsule, certain movements will be limited more than others. In the case of the shoulder, lateral rotation (placing the hand behind the neck) becomes more limited and painful than medial rotation (putting the hand behind the back). The rotation movements can be regained by trying to touch the fingers together behind the back (exercise 94). Joint play can also be regained by holding on to an object and leaning back to pull the shoulder along its length and apply traction. Alternatively, sit sideways on a dining chair and hang your arm over the chair back. Place a thick towel over the chair back to pad the armpit area. Grasp something in the hand to provide a traction force, and pull down on the stiff arm with the other arm to give overpressure (*see* fig 16.12(a)).

Tennis elbow

In tennis elbow, the muscle most commonly affected is the one that extends the wrist (extensor carpi radialis longus). This muscle will become tight and must be stretched by flexing the wrist while keeping the elbow

Figure 16.12 Self-traction in the shoulder joint: (a) hang arm over chair back

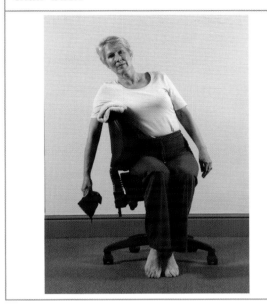

Figure 16.13 Stretching the extensor carpi radialis longus muscle in tennis elbow

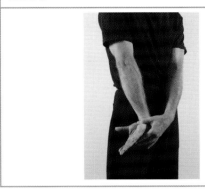

Tennis elbow often involves the nervous tissues traveling through the elbow. The upper limb tension test movements described in Chapter 15 are usually very relevant. Re-strengthening the forearm extensor muscles is also vital.

locked out. If the elbow is allowed to bend even slightly, the stretch will be taken off. A simple exercise is to stand facing a wall, and to straighten the elbow and keep it locked with pressure from the other hand. Place the back of the hand of the injured side against the wall and lean forwards to press the wrist into flexion (*see* exercise 68). Performed correctly, this stretch can be felt up the whole arm and into the elbow.

Because the extensor carpi radialis longus also abducts the wrist, a further stretch can be placed on the muscle by adducting the wrist at the same time as flexing it. This is achieved by standing with the arm by the side, pronating the forearm and flexing the wrist (*see* fig 16.13). Take hold of the hand and press the wrist into further flexion and adduction, pulling the wrist towards the little finger (ulnar deviation).

Wrist injury

Following a wrist injury, such as a severe sprain or fracture, most of the movements at the wrist will be limited. To regain these, three exercises are important. The first two are performed with the hand flat on a table top. Initially, the hand is placed palm down on the table surface, with the wrist crease at the table edge. The uninjured hand is placed on top of the injured one, and the elbow is moved up and down to produce flexion and extension of the wrist (*see* fig 16.14(a)). The leverage provided by the forearm, combined with the weight of the body provides overpressure at end-range for the static stretch.

For the second exercise, the hand is moved into the centre of the table so that the whole forearm is supported, and again the uninjured hand holds the injured one flat against the table surface. The elbow on the injured side is moved

Figure 16.14 Wrist mobility exercises

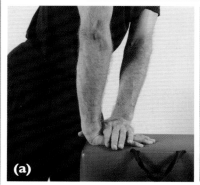 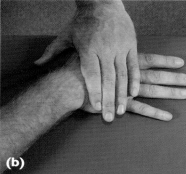 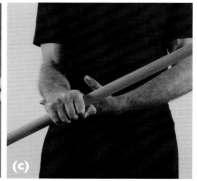

(a) (b) (c)

from side to side, sliding over the table surface to perform abduction and adduction of the injured wrist (*see* fig 16.14(b)). Finally, the arm is held at 90-degree flexion with the elbow close into the side of the body and the injured forearm supported by the cupped uninjured hand. A stick is held in the hand, and pronation and supination performed. Aim to move the stick into a horizontal position (*see* fig 16.14(c)).

Finger injuries

Finger injuries are common in many sports and are caused either through trauma, for example in martial arts and football, or from overuse, for example in rock climbing. Where swelling is profuse, movement can often become limited very quickly, so stretching is vital. As the structures of the hand and fingers are very delicate, the stretching should be applied 'little and often' as a general rule. Three or four shorter bouts per day are better than a single long bout.

The movements are flexion, extension, and abduction, all performed with manual overpressure. For flexion, the finger is bent to its maximal extent, and then gripped on the proximal and distal phalanx. Pressure is exerted to try to bring the finger tip to the underside of the knuckle. With extension, the movement must be isolated to each individual joint. One finger is placed proximal to the joint to fix it, while the other is placed distal to the joint to force the movement. For both of these movements, the exercise is best performed after soaking the hand and fingers in comfortably hot water for 15–20 minutes. Abduction is performed with the hand supported on a flat surface. The fingers are abducted and overpressure placed using two fingers of the opposite hand. The pressure is maintained for 20–30 seconds and then released.

Summary

- Inflammation shows as redness, swelling, heat and pain.
- Proliferation is the stage of tissue regeneration.
- During proliferation, dead tissue is removed by white blood cells and new tissue forms. Controlled movement is needed to encourage correct tissue placement.
- When injured, ligaments sprain and muscles strain.
- Stretching forms a vital part of injury recovery.

SPORT-SPECIFIC STRETCHING

17

Designing your own programme

In the majority of sports there is a central core of muscles that require stretching. Most sports involve some type of running action: this may be repeated running (marathon); single step running or lunging (badminton); or small bursts of speed (football). In each case the muscles used are similar, but the intensity of use and the range of motion will differ. While the running action forms the basis of motion, the throwing action frequently involves either a ball (throw and catch) or an implement used to strike an object (racquet or bat). Superimposed on these two basic sports movements are actions specific to the individual sports themselves. For example, the double-arm throwing action used in football differs considerably from the action of throwing the javelin, while the striking action of bat on ball in cricket is different from that of hitting a ball with a tennis racquet.

Therefore, to build up a comprehensive stretching programme for sports we need to choose exercises that cover both the core sports actions and the specific sports actions. By analysing which muscles are used in an action, we can estimate the patterns of muscle tightness that are likely to occur for each sport. Developing a stretching programme in this way can achieve two things. First, sports actions will be more efficient because we maintain a high range of motion. As we have seen on page 29, if a muscle is contracted from a comfortably stretched position, the amount of force achieved is greater than if a muscle is contracted from a shortened position. By stretching, we are therefore enhancing sports performance. Second, by preventing excessive shortening in general, and muscle imbalance in particular, we are maintaining optimal joint alignment. This provides a foundation for good biomechanics and balanced joint loading, increasing the likelihood of injury prevention.

> **Key point**: Movement analysis provides us with an accurate baseline upon which to build a stretching programme.

Movement analysis of core sports actions

Running

Running differs from walking in that when we walk we have at least one foot on the ground at all times; when we run we literally jump from foot to foot, so there is a stage when both feet are off the ground and the body is airborne. For this reason, running can be divided into two component phases, *stance* and *swing* (*see* fig 17.1). In the stance phase, the foot is on the ground and the body is decelerating. The muscles are working eccentrically to slow the body down and absorb shock through the whole of the lower limb. At the moment when the foot strikes the ground,

Figure 17.1 The running cycle (Norris 1998)

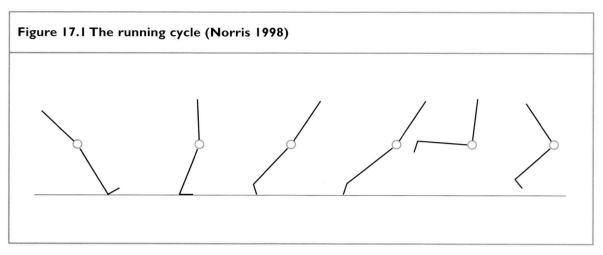

the body-weight is taken through the heel. As the body-weight moves forwards, the foot flattens to absorb the shock, and finally the foot pushes with the toes to accelerate the body once more and propel it forwards. The forward action signals the start of the swing phase when the foot is off the ground. The limb is now accelerating and being catapulted through the air.

During heel strike, the anterior tibial muscles work to stop the foot slapping down on the ground, while the posterior tibials stop the foot from flattening too much. Tightness in either of these two muscle groups can be a cause of shin pain in runners. In mid-stance the knee is bent slightly and the quadriceps work to provide the spring in the legs, while the hip abductors support the pelvis and prevent it dipping down at the side. Tightness in these muscles at this stage of running is one cause of pain at the side of the leg and knee (or 'runner's knee'). As the heel rises and we begin to push off from the floor, the hamstrings rapidly extend the hip while the calf muscles plantarflex the foot. Both provide the thrust in running. If either muscle is tight, it is more likely to tear during sudden lunging or sprinting actions. During the swing phase, the hip flexors lift the leg through. These muscles may become tight and therefore more susceptible

to injury, but usually any excessive tightness or shortness will affect the lumbar spine.

Stretches for running

Sports involving the running action will require calf, Achilles and anterior tibial stretches. In addition the hip flexors, hamstrings and quadriceps should be stretched, together with the abductors. Sprinting actions will require more attention to the hamstrings, while for kicking actions the rectus femoris will need stretching. Endurance running will need stretches for the ilio-tibial band (ITB) and anterior tibial muscles in particular, to protect against overuse friction injuries to these areas.

Throwing

In many sports the throwing mechanism is very similar. A javelin throw and an overhead shot in tennis may seem very different, but both have three phases (*see* fig 17.2).

Initially there is the cocking phase, in which the arm is held up and back in preparation for the strike. The shoulder is abducted and externally rotated, the elbow flexed and the wrist extended. This position stretches the anterior shoulder structures and shoulder rotators and

> **Figure 17.2 The throwing action: (a) The throwing action: (i) wind-up – athlete positions himself for the throw; (ii) cocking – lead leg moves forward, arm moves backwards stretching body; (iii) acceleration – body drives forwards leaving arm behind; (iv) deceleration – object released, elbow continues to extend and shoulder to internally rotate; (v) follow through – trunk and lead leg show eccentric activity to dissipate energy; (b) similarity of throwing action to tennis serve (Norris 1998)**

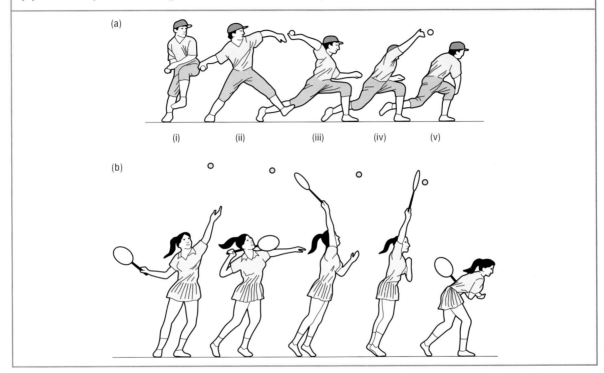

can place considerable stress on the medial ligament of the elbow. As the arm is pulled forwards into the striking position, it enters the acceleration phase. The body and shoulder lead the movement, coming forwards and leaving the arm behind, which pre-stretches the shoulder tissues. The shoulder flexors then contract rapidly with the shoulder rotators and elbow extensors to simultaneously bring the arm forwards and in. The acceleration phase takes place as a whipping action and so places considerable stress on the elbow structures. As the hand is flung forwards, the arm enters its final phase, the follow through. The object being thrown is released from the hand and the elbow extends rapidly. This places considerable stress on the bony knuckle of the ulna (olecranon process) as the elbow locks out.

Stretches for throwing

Sports involving any type of throwing action will require stretches to the anterior shoulder structures, the shoulder rotators and the elbow flexors. In addition, because of the single-arm nature of throwing, stretching must ensure symmetry between the two upper limbs.

Movement analysis of specific sports actions

To know which additional stretching exercises are required, we need to analyse a particular movement used in a sport to find out which muscles it is affecting.

It is usually the muscles stretched by large movement ranges that we are concerned with, because these will be the ones needing stretching exercises: when throwing the javelin, for example, the shoulder and elbow of the throwing arm travel through extreme ranges so they will need stretching. The amount particular muscles are used must also be noted; those used powerfully are likely to shorten and require additional stretching. For example, the pectorals and anterior deltoids are used powerfully when performing bench-press actions in weight training, so they tend to become very short.

Postures used in a sport are also a clue to the stretches that may be needed. Prolonged activity in a particular posture will cause the body to adapt by lengthening muscles on over-stretched joints, and shortening those other joints not moved through an adequate range. In cycling, for example, the stooped position of the thoracic spine can give rise to stiffness and pain in this area.

The movement analysis process may be divided into four stages.

- **Stage one**: Initially, we look at the movement and decide in which plane the movement mainly occurs (see fig 1.14, page 12). This will give us an idea of the types of movement used. Abduction and adduction occur in the frontal plane, flexion and extension in a sagittal plane, and rotation in a transverse plane.
- **Stage two**: Once we have an idea of the type of movement involved in an action, we must decide which joints are moving and which remain still. For example, in a trunk movement, is the hip moving as well? Does the pelvis move on the spine or on the hip, or both?
- **Stage three**: After the joints, we consider the muscles that would ordinarily work to bring about the actions we have seen, for example the muscles that flex the hip. We then need to determine if these muscles are actually working during the sporting action we are looking at, and to do this we must palpate (touch) the muscle.
- **Stage four**: Finally, the fact that a muscle is working during a movement does not necessarily mean that it warrants stretching. To determine this, we need to know the range of motion (see page 195). It is only when a muscle is taken through a greater range than normal (full outer- and full inner-range, rather than simply mid-range) that we need to stretch it.

> **Key point**: To analyse a movement, determine: (a) the plane of movement; (b) the joints moved; (c) the muscles stretched; and (d) the range of motion.

We will look at three examples from common sports to illustrate the movement analysis method: a football kick, a forehand shot in tennis and a golf swing when teeing off.

The football kick

When a kicking action is performed, the movement analysis is as follows:

- The movement occurs in both a sagittal plane and a frontal plane because the kick moves forwards and across the body.
- This movement will be flexion and adduction

of the hip, extension of the knee and plantarflexion of the ankle.

- Some transverse plane motion may also be seen as the trunk rotates on the standing leg.
- The muscles involved in this action would, therefore, be the hip flexors and adductors, knee extensors and ankle plantarflexors. In addition, the abductor muscles of the standing leg will stabilise the pelvis to stop it from dipping, and the trunk muscles will control the trunk rotation brought about by the momentum of the swinging leg.
- The range of motion of both the hip flexors and adductors is greater than normal, as is the range of the plantarflexors. The twisting of the spine would only be greater than normal in a less active individual who is beginning or returning to play.

The stretching exercises to choose, therefore, would be for the hip flexors, hip adductors (including gracilis) and calf muscles. Exercises 8, 9 and 22 would be appropriate.

The forehand in tennis

In an average tennis forehand shot, the movement analysis is as follows:

- The left leg steps across the right to bring the body to face right (right trunk rotation).
- The right hand is raised (abducted and extended) to shoulder level with the elbow and wrist partially extending.
- The foot action is one of dorsiflexion, stretching the calf.
- The combination of trunk rotation and shoulder abduction/extension is usually rapid, though not of extreme range.
- Stretching exercises for the chest and shoulder should, therefore, be combined with power training for this area. The calf/Achilles

and wrist extensors are taxed considerably in all racquet sports through repetitive actions, so they too will require stretching.

Exercise 91 is appropriate for the chest/shoulder, while exercises 9 and 68 are useful for the calf/achilles and wrist extensors.

The golf swing

In a typical golf swing (teeing off), the movement analysis is as follows:

- The body is angled forwards on the hips (pelvis anteriorly tilted on the hip) and the knees and hips are slightly flexed.
- The trunk is twisted (rotation) to the right on the semi-flexed leg.
- The arms are brought across the body to the right, raising the elbows to shoulder level and taking the hands over the right shoulder. To do this, the right shoulder externally rotates and the left internally rotates; these movements are reversed during the follow through.
- The trunk movement and the momentum of the combined body and club are taken through the semiflexed knee and considerable rotation occurs, slowly during the wind-up, and much more rapidly during the swing and follow through.
- The areas of concern are the combined movements at the trunk (flexion and rotation), which occur at speed and through considerable range, and the rotation at the knee. Both sets of movement are considerably greater than the normal movement ranges encountered in everyday life.

Trunk rotation stretches, pelvic tilt rehearsal and hip rotation movements are all important, with exercises 43 and 103 being appropriate. In addition, postural reeducation may be required if an individual angles the body forwards through trunk flexion alone, with little movement of the pelvis on the hip.

Summary

- Running and throwing are core skills in many sporting activities.

- There are four stages to movement analysis: establishing the plane of movement, finding which joints have moved, determining which muscles are working and finding the range of motion.

RECOMMENDED READING

Abdominal Training by Christopher M. Norris (A & C Black, London 1997)

Anatomy and Human Movement by N. Palastanga, D. Field and R. Soames (Butterworth Heinemann, Oxford 1994)

Back Stability by Christopher M. Norris (Human Kinetics, Champaign, Illinois 1999)

Bodytoning by Christopher M. Norris (A & C Black, London 2003)

Human Movement Explained by K. Jones and K. Barker (Butterworth Heinemann, Oxford 1996)

Joint Structure and Function (3rd edition) by P. K. Levangie and C. C. Norkin (F. A. Davies, Philadelphia 2001)

Muscles: Testing and Function by F. P. Kendall, E.K. McCreary and P. G. Provance (Williams and Wilkins, Baltimore 1993)

Neuromechanical Basis of Kinesiology (3rd edition) by R. M. Enoka (Human Kinetics, Champaign, Illinois 2002)

Sports Injuries, Diagnosis and Management (3rd edition) by Christopher M. Norris (Butterworth Heinemann, Oxford 2004)

The Complete Guide to Strength Training (2nd edition) by Anita Bean (A & C Black, London 2001)

REFERENCES

Adams, M. A., Hutton, W. C. and Stott, J. R. R. 1980, 'The resistance to flexion of the lumbar intervertebral joint', *Spine*, 5: 245–253

Astrand, P. O. and Rodahl, K. 1986, *Textbook of Work Physiology*, McGraw-Hill, Maidenhead

Bandy, W. D. and Irion, J. M. 1994, 'The effect of time on static stretch of the flexibility of the hamstring muscles', *Physical Therapy*, 74(9): 845–52

Barnard, H., Gardner, G. W., Diaco, N. V., MacAlpin, R. N. and Kattus, A. A., 1973, 'Cardiovascular responses to sudden strenuous exercise. Heart rate, blood pressure, and ECG', *Journal of Applied Physiology*, 34: 883–92

Bergh, U. 1980, 'Human power at subnormal body temperatures', *Acta Physiologica Scandinavia*, 478 (supplement): 1–39

Bergh, U. and Ekblom, B., 1979, 'Physical performance and peak aerobic power at different body temperatures', *Journal of Applied Physiology*, 46: 885–9

Butler, D. S., 1991, *Mobilisation of the Nervous System*, Churchill Livingstone, Edinburgh

Ekstrand, J., Gillquist, J., and Lilzedahl, S. S., 1983, 'Prevention of soccer injuries. Supervision by doctor and physiotherapist', *American Journal of Sports Medicine*, 11: 116–20

Enoka, R. M., 1994, Neuromechanical basis of kinesiology, *Human Kinetics*, Champaign, Illinois, USA

Etnyre, B. R. and Abraham, L. D., 1986, 'Gains in range of ankle dorsiflexion using three popular stretching techniques', *American Journal of Physical Medicine*, 65: 189–96

Fradkin, A. J., Gabbe, B. J and Cameron, P. A. (2006) Does warming up prevent injury in sport? The evidence from randomised controlled trials. *Journal of Science and Medicine in Sport*. 9(3): 214–220

Gleim, G. W., Stachenfeld, N. S. and Nicholas, J. A., 1990, 'The influence of flexibility on the ecconomy of walking and jogging', *Journal of Orthopaedic Research*, 8: 814–23

Godges, J. J., MacRae, H. and Longdon, C., 1989, 'The effects of two stretching procedures on hip range of motion and gait economy', *Journal of Orthopedic and Sports Physical Therapy* 10(9): 350–7

Halbertsma, J. A., van Bolhuis, A. L. and Gloehen, L. N., 1996, *Archives of Physical Medicine and Rehabilitation*, 77: 688–692

Johns, R. J. and Wright, V., 1992, 'Relative importance of various tissues in joint stiffness', *Journal of Applied Physiology*, 17: 824–8

LaBan, M. M., 1962, 'Collagen tissue: implications of its response to stress in vitro', *Archives of Physical Medicine and Rehabilitation*, 43: 461–6

Li, Y., McClure, P. W. and Pratt, N., 1996, 'The effect of hamstring muscle stretching on standing posture and on lumbar and hip motions during forward bending', *Physical Therapy*, 76: 836–45

Magnusson, S. P., Simonsen, E. B. and Kjaer, M., 1996, 'Biomechanical responses to repeated stretches in human hamstring muscle in vitro', *American Journal of Sports Medicine*, 24(5): 622–8

McNair, P. J. and Stanley, S. N., 1996, 'Effect of passive stretching and jogging on the series elastic muscle stiffness and range of motion of the ankle joint', *British Journal of Sports Medicine*, 30: 313–8

Millar, A. P., 1976, 'An early stretching routine of calf muscle strains', *Medicine and Science in Sports and Exercise*, 22(3): 632–41

Moore, M. A. and Kukulka, C. G., 1991, 'Depression of Hoffman reflexes following voluntary contraction and implications for proprioceptive neuromuscular facilitation therapy', *Physical Therapy*, 71: 321–33

Nelson, A. G., Kokkonen, J., and Arnall, D. A. (2005) Acute muscle stretching inhibits muscle strength endurance performance. *Journal of Strength and Conditioning Research*. 19(2): 338–343

Nicol, C., Komi, P. V. and Horita, T., 1996, 'Reduced stretch–reflex sensitivity after exhausting stretch–shortening cycle exercise', *European Journal of Applied Physiology*, 72: 401–9

Norris, C. M., 1998, *Sports Injuries. Diagnosis and Management*, Butterworth Heinemann, London

Rosenbaum, D. and Henning, E. M., 1995, 'The influence of stretching and warm-up exercises on Achilles tendon reflex activity', *Journal of Sports Science*, 15: 481–4

Safran, M. R., Garrett, W. E., Seaber, A. V., Glisson, R. R. and Ribbecsk, B. M., 1988, 'The role of warm-up in muscular injury prevention', *American Journal of Sports Medicine*, 16(2)

Shrier, I. (2004) Does stretching improve performance? A systematic and critical review of the literature. *Clinical Journal of Sports Medicine.* 14(5): 267–273

Sullivan, M. K., Dejulia, J. J. and Worrell, T. W., 1992, 'Effect of pelvic position and stretching method on hamstring muscle flexibility', *Medicine and Science in Sports and Exercise*, 24: 1383–9

Taylor, D. C., Dalton, J., Seaber, A. V, and Garrett, W. E., 1990, 'The viscoelastic properties of muscle-tendon units', *American Journal of Sports Medicine*, 18: 300–9

Thomas, J. R. and Nelson, J. K., 1990, second edition, Research Methods in Physical Activity, *Human Kinetics*, Champaign, Illinois, USA.

Warren, C. G., Lehmann, J. F. and Koblanski, J. N., 1971, 'Elongation of rat tail tendon: effect of load and temperature', *Archives of Physical Medicine and Rehabilitation*, 51: 465–74

Webright, W. G., Randolph, B. J. and Perrin, D. H., 1997, 'Comparison of nonballistic active knee extension in neural slump position and static techniques on hamstring flexibility', *Journal of Orthopedic and Sports Physical Therapy*, 26: 7–13

Witvrouw, E., Mahieu, N., Danneels, L., and McNair, P. (2004) Stretching and injury prevention: an obscure relationship. *Sports Medicine* 34(7): 443–439

INDEX OF EXERCISES

INDEX

ALSO AVAILABLE

The Complete Guide to Sports Massage – 2nd edition
Tim Paine

Sports massage is the skilled manipulation of soft tissue for the relief and treatment of muscle soreness and pain, the maintenance of muscle balance and improved flexibility, and enhanced rehabilitation from injury.

The Complete Guide to Sports Massage is a comprehensive manual packed with jargon-free information and practical tips, and includes principles and techniques of massage (including step-by-step instructions), injury management and post-massage care, and practical guidance on working at a sports event.

Fully updated in full colour for the new edition, with new photographs demonstrating massage technique throughout, and clear and helpful anatomical illustrations, this is the definitive practical handbook for students of sports therapy and anyone wanting a performance advantage.

Available from all good bookshops and online. For more information on this and other A&C Black Sport & Fitness titles, please go to www.acblack.com

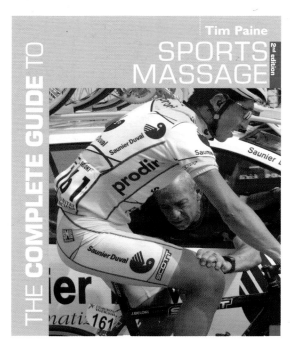